Autism and Child Psychopathology Series

Series Editor:
Johnny L. Matson
Department of Psychology
Louisiana State University
Baton Rouge, LA, USA

For further volumes:
http://www.springer.com/series/8665

Giulio E. Lancioni · Jeff Sigafoos
Mark F. O'Reilly · Nirbhay N. Singh

Assistive Technology

Interventions for Individuals with Severe/ Profound and Multiple Disabilities

Springer

Giulio E. Lancioni
Department of Neuroscience and Sense Organs, University of Bari
Bari, Italy

Mark F. O'Reilly
Department of Special Education
University of Texas at Austin
The Meadows Center for Preventing Educational Risk
Austin, TX, USA

Jeff Sigafoos
Victoria University of Wellington
School of Educational Psychology & Pedagogy, Karori Campus
Wellington, New Zealand

Nirbhay N. Singh
American Health and Wellness Institute
Raleigh, NC, USA

ISSN 2192-922X ISSN 2192-9238 (electronic)
ISBN 978-1-4614-4228-8 ISBN 978-1-4614-4229-5 (eBook)
DOI 10.1007/978-1-4614-4229-5
Springer New York Heidelberg Dordrecht London

Library of Congress Control Number: 2012938480

Printed on acid-free paper

Springer is part of Springer Science+Business Media (www.springer.com)

To our families

Preface

This book summarizes research activity directed at assessing the value and impact of various types of assistive technologies for enhancing the abilities and overall quality of life for persons with severe/profound and multiple disabilities. The research areas reviewed in the various chapters of the book largely correspond to the main research activities of the authors. Thus, research is reviewed that covers the use of microswitches for increasing independence and the use of speech-generating devices for improving communication interactions with others. We also review studies that have focused on the use of assistive technologies for promoting occupational outcomes and reducing problematic forms of behavior.

The aim of the book is to provide readers with an up-to-date picture of the scientific evidence available in the areas covered. The studies reviewed in each chapter were carefully selected to represent the best available evidence. Within each chapter, this evidence is summarized in terms of the technological devices used, the intervention programs applied to teach the use of those devices, the persons involved in the intervention programs, and the outcomes of the intervention programs. We also provide summative conclusions of the evidence and include a discussion of areas of future need and development. This book is intended to guide evidence-based practice in the field and offer direct support to the practitioner. Practitioners will learn how the technology can be employed, what types of interventions have been used with each type of technology, and the outcomes that can be expected.

The book also serves as an occasion to thank (a) the many participants involved in our studies, their families, and the staff personnel responsible for their daily programs; (b) the researchers and technical experts (engineers) who have made the studies possible; and (c) the organizations that have supported our research initiatives. With regard to the researchers, we would like to single out the extensive contribution of Doretta Oliva. With regard to the technical experts, we would like to acknowledge the continuous input of Domenico Bellini, Sandro Bracalente, and

Gianluigi Montironi. In terms of organizations, we want to emphasize the lasting positive role of the Lega F. D'Oro Research Center, Osimo, Italy; the Autism Treatment Centers of Dallas and San Antonio, Texas; and our respective institutions: University of Bari, Italy; Victoria University of Wellington, New Zealand; The University of Texas at Austin; and the American Health and Wellness Institute.

Contents

About the Authors

Giulio E. Lancioni, Ph.D., is Professor in the Department of Neuroscience and Sense Organs, University of Bari, Italy. He also spent many years at the Department of Psychology, University of Leiden, the Netherlands. His research interests include development and assessment of assistive technologies, training of social and occupational skills, and evaluation of strategies for examining preference and choice of individuals with severe/profound intellectual and multiple disabilities (including post-coma persons in a minimally conscious state and persons with Alzheimer's disease). He has published widely in these areas and serves in the editorial board of several international journals concerned with these topics.

Jeff Sigafoos, Ph.D., is Professor in the School of Educational Psychology and Pedagogy, Victoria University of Wellington, New Zealand. Prior to this position, he held appointments at the University of Queensland, the University of Sydney, and The University of Texas at Austin. His research interests include communication assessment and intervention for individuals with developmental and physical disabilities, educational programming for children with autism spectrum disorders, and the assessment and treatment of problem behavior in individuals with developmental and physical disabilities. He has published widely in these areas and is the Editor of *Developmental Neurorehabilitation* and Coeditor-in-Chief of *Evidence-Based Communication Assessment and Intervention.*

Mark F. O'Reilly, Ph.D., holds the Mollie Villeret Davis Professorship in Learning Disabilities and is Professor of Special Education in the Department of Special Education at The University of Texas at Austin. He lectured in the Department of Psychology at University College Dublin, Ireland, prior to his current appointment. His research interests include assessment and treatment of severe challenging behavior in individuals with autism spectrum disorders and other developmental disorders, design and evaluation of assistive technology to support individuals with severe/profound and multiple disabilities, and communication/social skills interventions for individuals with intellectual disabilities. He is the Editor-in-Chief of the *Journal of Developmental and Physical Disabilities.*

Nirbhay N. Singh, Ph.D., is the Chief Learning and Development Officer at the American Health and Wellness Institute, Raleigh, North Carolina. He was Professor of Psychiatry, Pediatrics, and Psychology at the Virginia Commonwealth University School of Medicine and Director of the Commonwealth Institute for Family Studies, Richmond, Virginia, prior to his current appointment. His research interests include behavioral and psychopharmacological treatments of individuals with disabilities, assistive technology for supporting individuals with severe/profound and multiple disabilities, and mindfulness. He is the Editor-in-Chief of the *Journal of Child and Family Studies* and *Mindfulness* and Editor of the book series *Mindfulness in Behavioral Health.*

Chapter 1
Defining Assistive Technology and the Target Populations

Abstract This chapter introduces the notion of assistive technology and provides illustrative examples of its use with schoolchildren with typical intellectual functioning and persons with severe/profound and multiple disabilities. This chapter also provides a brief summary of the intervention areas and forms of assistive technology covered by the subsequent chapters in this book. These areas and technologies concern the following: interaction with the environment and control of stimulation through microswitches (Chap. 2); communication through speech-generating devices (SGDs) (Chap. 3); academic, work, and leisure activity engagement through an array of technology-based programs (Chap. 4); independent travel within indoor areas through orientation systems (Chap. 5); ambulation through treadmills, walkers, and microswitches or a robot (Chap. 6); and reduction of problem behaviors through SGDs, microswitches, or microswitch clusters (Chap. 7).

Introduction

Assistive technology refers to a variety of devices (and services related to their use) aimed at helping persons with disabilities and special education/rehabilitation needs to function better within their daily context and achieve a higher quality of life. Specifically, assistive technology encompasses multiple resources (capable of providing different forms of practical support), which are expected to produce important behavioral and social benefits for the users by reducing the negative impact of their disabilities and related (problematic) conditions (Bauer et al. 2011; Brown et al. 2009; Reichle 2011; Shih 2011). The first requirement for the realization of this goal is that the users (i.e., the persons with disabilities) receive the types of assistive technologies that are best suited to their characteristics, their tasks, and their environments (Bauer et al. 2011; Borg et al. 2011). The mere provision of assistive technology, even if carefully matched as mentioned above, however, may not be sufficient to guarantee a positive outcome. Such an outcome may become

G.E. Lancioni et al., *Assistive Technology: Interventions for Individuals with Severe/Profound and Multiple Disabilities*, Autism and Child Psychopathology Series, DOI 10.1007/978-1-4614-4229-5_1,

much more likely if one adds to the provision of technology an explicit and carefully designed intervention aimed at ensuring that the persons learn how to use it effectively.

In light of the above, one can argue that the increased production and availability of new technologies to assist persons with disabilities would have an increasingly relevant role (i.e., progressively wider practical implications) if paralleled by effective interventions to enable those persons to make successful use of such technologies (Burne et al. 2011; Rispoli et al. 2010). This link between technologies and interventions could be seen as a new, emerging specialty field that integrates rehabilitation engineering with rehabilitation psychology, behavior analysis, and special education. The fact that the number of devices developed and made available has grown consistently over the years can be taken as (a) a sign of an increasing attention to the rights of persons with special education/rehabilitation needs (i.e., a growing recognition that these persons must not be left behind) and (b) an attempt to provide these persons the opportunity to be involved meaningfully in a gradually more inclusive society (Borg et al. 2011; Parette et al. 2010). In practice, these devices are conceived with the view of enabling persons with serious limitations in their developmental, communication, and/or occupational perspectives to improve their general participation opportunities, that is, to gain greater access to their daily environment and related choice events, with important personal and social implications (Collins et al. 1991; Moisey 2007; Moisey and van de Keere 2007; Ripat and Woodgate 2011; Scherer et al. 2011).

Two large groups of persons have received particular attention in terms of assistive technology, namely, (a) students with combinations of motor or sensory-motor and communication disabilities and typical or nearly typical level of intellectual functioning, and (b) persons with severe/profound intellectual disabilities or combinations of motor or sensory-motor impairment and intellectual disabilities or consciousness disorders. Assistive technology devices that may be employed within educational (school) programs to help the former group of persons include among others (a) modified (e.g., expanded) keyboards aimed at allowing the persons to press the keys and enter the letters so as to write successfully, (b) electronic pointing instruments used in substitution of the mouse and possibly of the keyboard, (c) on-screen keyboards (keyboard emulators) that often include the scanning function to allow the persons to choose the keyboard keys with a simple response that might be a minimal movement of any part of the body, (d) text-to-speech synthesizer that allow the persons to enter written text information and translate it into speech that the persons can use to communicate with relevant people in the environment (Burne et al. 2011; Handley 2009; Hertzum and Hornbaek 2010; Lancioni et al. 2009; Matias et al. 1996; Shih 2011; Shih and Shih 2010).

Assistive technology devices, that may be employed within programs for the latter group of persons (i.e., those with intellectual disabilities or consciousness disorders often combined with motor and/or communication impairments), include among others (a) microswitches aimed at allowing the persons to access (control the occurrence of) environmental stimulation with minimal responses, (b) speech-generating devices (SGDs) allowing the persons to translate their simple motor responses into the production/utterance of verbal messages (requests), (c) spatial orientation systems aimed at helping the persons to reach target places within their indoor areas through the use of auditory or visual direction cues or through corrective feedback, (d) computer-aided instruction systems aimed at providing verbal or pictorial cues to support the persons through the performance of multistep activities, and (e) microswitch clusters to strengthen adaptive responses and inhibit problematic behavior (Furniss et al. 1999; Lancioni et al. 2007, 2008; Rispoli et al. 2010; Sigafoos et al. 2009; Thunberg et al. 2007). In the past, before the assistive technologies were available, these persons were generally deemed as dependent on staff care and stimulation. With the development and availability of the assistive technologies, these persons are considered capable of achieving relevant levels of self-determination and active engagement, with control of their stimulation input and improvement of their mood (Lancioni et al. 2005, 2008).

Assistive Technology for School Settings and Students with Typical Intellectual Functioning

An illustrative example of assistive technology for students with typical intellectual functioning, which we may describe here in terms of its basic characteristics and possible impact, concerns a keyboard emulator with a scanning function. The scanning function is typically combined with a virtual keyboard appearing on a computer screen. Such a device is usually designed for persons who have serious difficulties using real keyboards including those modified with the aim of facilitating their use (i.e., modified to help persons who have limited control of their hand and finger movements). The scanning may initially concern the keyboard rows, one at a time. Following the person's response in relation to a row, the scanning may concern the single keys of that row, one at a time. The person's response to one key would write the corresponding letter/symbol on the upper part of the computer screen and restart the scanning of the rows. The person's response is carried out with a single input tool, such as a touch-pad sensor that can be activated through a simple (nonspecific) hand movement. In a recent study by Lancioni et al. (2009), for example, the technology included a commercially available scanning keyboard emulator (WiViK by Prentke Romich Company, Wooster, OH, USA), which appeared on a computer screen and was combined with a voice-detecting sensor serving as input tool. The sensor could be activated with a brief vocal emission, that is, with a response considered to be suitable for both participants (two schoolchildren) because they could perform it fairly rapidly, reliably, and without much effort. The keyboard emulator appeared in the lower half of the computer screen. When the children responded (with a vocal emission) to a keyboard row, scanning continued on groups of keys of the row selected. The children's responding to a group led to the scanning of the single keys of it with the possibility of selecting one of them and writing the corresponding symbol (i.e., as mentioned above).

Assistive Technology for Programs Involving Persons with Intellectual Disabilities or Consciousness Disorders

A first illustrative example of assistive technology, which may be described within this area, is the combined use of a microswitch and an SGD for post-coma persons with extensive neuromotor impairment and minimally conscious state. These persons are usually exposed to general forms of stimulation chosen by the rehabilitation staff and do not have the possibility of accessing stimulation on their own or of making requests of any type, given their widely compromised functioning situation (Lancioni et al. 2010a; Magee 2007; Zhu et al. 2009). The use of a microswitch would allow them to activate one or more sources of stimulation on an independent manner, that is, at their preferred times and according to their preferred frequencies, via a simple/affordable response. The use of an SGD would allow them to call a caregiver for requesting attention or particular forms of stimulation/interaction, thus increasing the level of input and restoring emotional and communication ties.

In a recent study by Lancioni et al. (2009), for example, a man was provided with an adapted optic microswitch that he could activate through eye blinks and a new (custom-made) SGD that he could activate through finger movements. Two blinks occurring within a 2-s interval were required to activate the optic microswitch. Each microswitch activation allowed him to listen to a brief period of preferred music. The SGD involved a cylinder-like device, which was fixed inside the man's hand and had two sensitive sections at the outer sides (i.e., the section of the device corresponding to the little finger and the one corresponding to the index finger). Activation of one of the sensitive sections caused the occurrence of a verbal call for the man's mother. Activation of the other sensitive section caused the occurrence of a verbal call for a research assistant who had long familiarized with him. Each one of the two (mother and research assistant) would have a specific form of interaction with the man for a brief interval of time.

A second illustrative example of assistive technology is represented by a computer-aided system that relies on a palmtop computer with a color screen. Such a system is easily portable and can help persons with severe intellectual disabilities perform daily activities by providing them pictorial instruction cues for the single steps of those activities. These persons are known to have difficulties managing the performance of relevant activities and to remain largely passive and dependent on staff's direct supervision, with negative implications for their occupational opportunities, their constructive interactions within the environment, and their social status (Brown et al. 2009; Friedman et al. 2009). The system would be easy for the persons to use. They would only need to make a simple response such as pressing a key to get the first/next pictorial instruction in the sequence. The pictorial instructions, moreover, would be interspersed with pictorial representations of positive (reinforcing) events such as the caregiver providing social approval or tangible items. These latter pictorial representations would be expected to ensure the persons' motivation to maintain continuity in seeking instructions and performing the related activity steps. To minimize errors and program misuses, one could develop few simple insurance conditions concerning, among others, the availability and change of instructions.

The evaluation of a similar form of computer-aided system was reported by Lancioni et al. (2000). The study included six adults whose level of intellectual functioning was rated in the severe disability range. The system involved an IBM 110 palmtop computer, electronic circuitry, an auditory output box, and a vibration box. The system had a single key that the participants were to press to cause the occurrence of a new pictorial instruction on the computer screen. The pictorial instructions referred to specific steps of the task at hand or to a reinforcing event. The latter types of instructions (i.e., those concerning reinforcing events) were sporadic and served to motivate the participants' performance. The participants carried with them either one of the aforementioned boxes (producing auditory or vibration output). Those boxes would provide them with prompting in case they failed to return to the computer and ask for a new instruction within a preset interval from the previous request. The system was also equipped with a latency function. This ensured that repeated key press responses would not cause accidental (erroneous) change of the pictorial instruction on the screen.

Assistive Technology Areas and Devices Touched in the Following Chapters

Each of the next six chapters (i.e., Chaps. 2, 3, 4, 5, 6 and 7) of this book concerns specific areas of intervention and related forms of assistive technology for persons with severe/profound and multiple disabilities. The chapters provide reviews of the literature available in the areas covered so as to present the reader with an illustrative picture of the intervention strategies and objectives, of the characteristics of the persons involved, of the assistive technology devices employed, and of the results obtained. The first of those six chapters (i.e., Chap. 2) concerns intervention efforts focused on helping persons with extensive physical impairment and other (e.g., intellectual and communication) disabilities to develop constructive interactions with their surroundings (Holburn et al. 2004; Lancioni et al. 2008). The main form of assistive technology adopted for persons with these characteristics consists of microswitches. Microswitch-based programs include three basic components, that is, an electronic control system, one or more microswitches, and environmental stimuli connected to the electronic control system. The person's activation of a microswitch triggers the electronic control system that turns on specific environmental stimuli for brief periods of time. Microswitches can be commercially available or experimental. The simultaneous availability of multiple microswitches allows the person to choose among different responses and stimulus sets (Lancioni et al. 2008, 2010a).

Chapter 3 concerns the use of SGDs, that is, assistive technology instruments that can be programmed to produce different types of verbal outputs in relation to nonverbal responses of the participants (see above). Those instruments represent forms of alternative communication technology for persons with communication impairment, that is, persons who are able to emit only largely unintelligible speech, have lost speech and communication abilities, or have never developed sufficient speech and language/communication abilities. Based on the characteristics and needs of the participants, the objectives of the intervention efforts vary and the characteristics of the technology may also differ. In general, the intervention efforts concern (a) the establishment of requesting skills (e.g., the persons are enabled to use the technology to verbalize requests of preferred items and activities), (b) the establishment of responses that allow the individual to communicate a desire to escape from or avoid nonpreferred objects and activities, and (c) establishment of socially oriented communication responses aimed at recruiting the attention of a listener or at initiating forms of conversation. SGDs vary from simple tools producing a brief prerecorded message to highly sophisticated computer technologies generating multiple and complex utterances via speech synthesis technology (Rispoli et al. 2010; Sigafoos et al. 2009).

Chapter 4 concerns the use of assistive technology for promoting academic, work, and leisure activities. The first part of the chapter analyzes studies that used technology solutions to enable writing by individuals who could not use standard implements, such as pens and standard computer keyboards, because of their multiple disabilities. The second part of the chapter analyzes studies that used technology to teach individuals to engage in occupational and vocational tasks. These studies used a variety of unsophisticated and sophisticated technology solutions for the presentation of instructions. Those instructions relied on picture prompts, object or tactile prompts, self-operated audio prompts, self-instruction prompts, video modeling and video prompts, palmtop-based job aids, and electronic control devices. The third part of the chapter analyzes studies on leisure skills that used technology to provide individuals access to different classes of leisure activities, that is, enabled them to access a variety of preferred stimulation and taught them to operate standard or adapted leisure modalities (e.g., radio, television, portable media player, and a computer for e-mail) and an electronic messaging system.

Chapter 5 concerns the use of assistive technology to help persons with orientation problems travel within indoor areas (i.e., their living and occupational contexts). Different orientation systems are available to respond to the requirements of persons with different characteristics. Persons who present with blindness or minimal residual vision and a very limited notion of space with virtually no orientation abilities may need very substantial help. Consequently, they would perform better with a system that does not require much initiative and self-direction from them (Lancioni et al. 2007). Such a system provides direction cues, that is, cues that guide the person's travel by marking/specifying the space leading to the destination (Lancioni et al. 2007, 2010b). The cues consist of buzzer-like sounds, verbal messages, and visual cues (lights). Persons who have functional vision and/or possess a general notion of the spatial reality within which they travel are able to benefit from a system that is less intrusive than the one mentioned above (i.e., the one using direction cues). This less intrusive system does not use direction cues, but rather employ corrective feedback. In practice, the system only intervenes if the person loses the correct direction. In that case, a feedback is presented to inform the persons that he or she has to change direction. The feedback lasts until the person has found the correct direction. At that point, he or she can start walking again.

Chapter 6 concerns the use of different technology-based approaches to support and promote walking. Those approaches are based on the notion of experience-dependent plasticity, which suggests that the way to improve a person's ambulatory behavior is to allow that person to practice it. The most popular technology-based approach is the one that relies on the use of treadmills generally combined with partial body weight support (Damiano and DeJong 2009). The strategy of supporting the participants' body weight (e.g., through a harness) is considered essential to facilitate their stepping responses particularly when the motor impairment is extensive or the motor condition is largely immature. A second technology-based approach is the one that combines the use of walker devices with microswitches. The walkers can be provided with supporting features that help facilitate postural control and partial weight lifting (Lancioni et al. 2005). The microswitches allow the monitoring of the participants' stepping responses and ensure the automatic delivery of brief periods of preferred environmental stimulation contingent on those responses. A third technology-based approach concerns the use of a robot, which provides the participants with physical support to ensure their balance and with guidance to walk to different destinations (Lancioni et al. 1997).

Chapter 7 concerns the use of assistive technology to reduce problem behavior. The intervention programs differ according to whether they are used to treat problem behavior that is maintained by escape from demands, access to attention or tangible items, or is self-stimulatory in nature. When the behavior is maintained by escape, the participants can be provided with an augmentative communication device (i.e., an SGD) and taught to use this technology to communicate a desire to terminate demands (Durand 1999). Demand termination can serve as a reinforcing event and establish the appropriate use of the device to make the request. The problem behavior is typically ignored during the program. When the behavior is maintained by attention or tangible items, the participant can be provided with an SGD, which is programmed to emit verbal requests for those events when triggered. When the behavior is self-stimulatory, the intervention can rely on different uses of microswitch technology. For example, it can resort to the use of (a) microswitches that produce positive stimulation when an adaptive behavior, alternative to self-stimulation, occurs and (b) microswitch clusters where an adaptive response (monitored by one microswitch) produces positive stimulation only when the self-stimulatory response (monitored by the second microswitch) does not occur (Cooper et al. 2009; Lancioni et al. 2008).

References

Bauer, S. M., Elsaesser, L.-J., & Arthanat, S. (2011). Assistive technology device classification based upon the World Health Organization's, International Classification of Functioning, Disability and Health (ICF). *Disability and Rehabilitation: Assistive Technology, 6*, 243–259.

Borg, J., Larson, S., & Östegren, P. O. (2011). The right to assistive technology: For whom, for what, and by whom? *Disability and Society, 26*, 151–167.

Brown, R. I., Schalock, R. L., & Brown, I. (2009). Quality of life: Its application to persons with intellectual disabilities and their families – introduction and overview. *Journal of Policy and Practice in Intellectual Disabilities, 6*, 2–6.

Burne, B., Knafelc, V., Melonis, M., & Heyn, P. C. (2011). The use and application of assistive technology to promote literacy in early childhood: A systematic review. *Disability and Rehabilitation: Assistive Technology, 6*, 207–213.

Collins, B. C., Gast, D. L., Wolery, M., Holcombe, A., & Leatherby, J. G. (1991). Constant time delay to teach self-feeding to young students with severe/profound handicaps: Evidence of limited effectiveness. *Journal of Developmental and Physical Disabilities, 3*, 157–179.

Cooper, S.-A., Smiley, E., Jackson, A., Finlayson, J., Allan, L. M., Mantry, D., & Morrison, J. (2009). Adults with intellectual disabilities: prevalence, incidence and remission of aggressive behavior and related factors. *Journal of Intellectual Disability Research, 53*, 217–232.

Damiano, D. L., & DeJong, S. L. (2009). A systematic review of the effectiveness of treadmill training and body weight support in pediatric rehabilitation. *Journal of Neurologic Physical Therapy, 33*, 27–44.

Durand, V. M. (1999). Functional communication training using assistive devices: Recruiting natural communities of reinforcement. *Journal of Applied Behavior Analysis, 32*, 247–267.

Friedman, B., Wamsley, B. R., Liebel, D. V., Saad, Z. B., & Eggert, G. M. (2009). Patient satisfaction, empowerment, and health and disability status effects of a disease management-health promotion nurse intervention among medicare beneficiaries with disabilities. *The Gerontolosgist, 49*, 778–792.

Furniss, F., Ward, A., Lancioni, G., Rocha, N., Cunha, B., Seedhouse, P., Morato, P., & Waddell, N. (1999). A palmtop-based job aid for workers with severe intellectual disabilities. *Technology and Disability, 10*, 53–67.

Handley, Z. (2009). Is text-to-speech synthesis ready for use in computer-assisted language learning? *Speech Communication, 51*, 906–919.

Hertzum, M., & Hornbaek, K. (2010). How age affects pointing with mouse and touchpad: A comparison of young, adult, and elderly users. *International Journal of Human Computer Interaction, 26*, 703–734.

Holburn, S., Nguyen, D., & Vietze, P. M. (2004). Computer-assisted learning for adults with profound multiple disabilities. *Behavioral Interventions, 19*, 25–37.

Lancioni, G. E., Bosco, A., Olivetti Belardinelli, M., Singh, N. N., O'Reilly, M. F., & Sigafoos, J. (2010a). An overview of intervention options for promoting adaptive behavior of persons with acquired brain injury and minimally conscious state. *Research in Developmental Disabilities, 31*, 1121–1134.

Lancioni, G. E., O'Reilly, M. F., Seedhouse, P., Furniss, F., & Cunha, B. (2000). Promoting independent task performance by persons with severe developmental disabilities through a new computer-aided system. *Behavior Modification, 24*, 724–741.

Lancioni, G. E., O'Reilly, M. F., Singh, N. N., Sigafoos, J., Oliva, D., Antonucci, M., Tota, A., & Basili, G. (2008). Microswitch-based programs for persons with multiple disabilities: An overview of some recent developments. *Perceptual and Motor Skills, 106*, 355–370.

Lancioni, G. E., O'Reilly, M. F., Singh, N. N., Sigafoos, J., Oliva, D., Bracalente, S., & Montironi, G. (2007). Orientation systems to support indoor travel by persons with multiple disabilities: Technical aspects and application issues. *Technology and Disability, 19*, 1–6.

Lancioni, G. E., Oliva, D., & O'Reilly, M. F. (1997). Ambulation, object manipulation, and multiple disabilities: Extending the applicability of a robot. *Journal of Visual Impairment & Blindness, 91*, 53–60.

Lancioni, G. E., Singh, N. N., O'Reilly, M. F., Campodonico, F., Piazzolla, G., Scalini, L., & Oliva, D. (2005). Impact of favorite stimuli automatically delivered on step responses of persons with multiple disabilities during their use of walker devices. *Research in Developmental Disabilities, 26*, 71–76.

Lancioni, G. E., Singh, N. N., O'Reilly, M. F., Sigafoos, J., Alberti, G., Scigliuzzo, F., Signorino, M., Oliva, D., Smaldone, A., & La Martire, M. L. (2010b). Persons with multiple disabilities use orientation technology to find room entrances during indoor traveling. *Research in Developmental Disabilities, 31*, 1577–1584.

Lancioni, G. E., Singh, N. N., O'Reilly, M. F., Sigafoos, J., Green, V., Chiapparino, C., Stasolla, F., & Oliva, D. (2009). A voice-detecting sensor and a scanning keyboard emulator to support word writing by two boys with extensive motor disabilities. *Research in Developmental Disabilities, 30*, 203–209.

Magee, W. L. (2007). Music as a diagnostic tool in low awareness states: Considering limbic responses. *Brain Injury, 21*, 593–599.

Matias, E., MacKenzie, I. S., & Buxton, W. (1996). One-handed touch typing on a QWERTY keyboard. *Human Computer Interaction, 11*, 1–27.

Moisey, S. D. (2007). The Inclusive Libraries Initiative: Enhancing the access of persons with developmental disabilities to information and communication technology. *Developmental Disabilities Bulletin, 35*, 56–71.

Moisey, S., & van de Keere, R. (2007). Inclusion and the Internet: Teaching adults with developmental disabilities to use information and communication technology. *Developmental Disabilities Bulletin, 35*, 72–102.

Parette, H. P., Meadan, H., Doubet, S., & Hess, J. (2010). Supporting families of young children with disabilities using technology. *Education and Training in Autism and Developmental Disabilities, 45*, 552–565.

Reichle, J. (2011). Evaluating assistive technology in the education of persons with severe disabilities. *Journal of Behavioral Education, 20*, 77–85.

Ripat, J., & Woodgate, R. (2011). The intersection of culture, disability and assistive technology. *Disability and Rehabilitation: Assistive Technology, 6*, 87–96.

Rispoli, M. J., Franco, J. H., van der Meer, L., Lang, R., & Camargo, S. P. H. (2010). The use of speech generating devices in communication interventions for individuals with developmental disabilities: A review of the literature. *Developmental Neurorehabilitation, 13*, 276–293.

Scherer, M. J., Craddock, G., & Mackeogh, T. (2011). The relationship of personal factors and subjective well-being to the use of assistive technology devices. *Disability and Rehabilitation, 33*, 811–817.

Shih, C.-H. (2011). Assisting people with developmental disabilities to improve computer pointing efficiency through multiple mice and automatic pointing assistive programs. *Research in Developmental Disabilities, 32*, 1736–1744.

Shih, C.-H., & Shih, C.-T. (2010). Development of an integrated pointing device driver for the disabled. *Disability and Rehabilitation. Assistive Technology, 5*, 351–358.

Sigafoos, J., Green, V. A., Payne, D., Son, S.-H., O'Reilly, M., & Lancioni, G. E. (2009). A comparison of picture exchange and speech generating devices: Acquisition, preference, and effects on social interaction. *AAC: Augmentative and Alternative Communication, 25*, 99–109.

Thunberg, G., Ahlsén, E., & Sandberg, A. D. (2007). Children with autistic spectrum disorders and speech-generating devices: Communication in different activities at home. *Clinical Linguistics & Phonetics, 21*, 457–479.

Zhu, J., Wu, X., Gao, L., Mao, Y., Zhong, P., Tang, W., & Zhou, L. (2009). Cortical activity after emotional visual stimulation in minimally conscious state patients. *Journal of Neurotrauma, 26*, 677–688.

Chapter 2
Use of Microswitches in Habilitation Programs

Abstract This chapter provides an overview of studies using microswitches for promoting adaptive/positive engagement of persons with profound and multiple disabilities. For practical (presentation) reasons, the studies are divided into several groups based on the responses targeted and the microswitches employed. A first group concerns studies that targeted a single typical response (e.g., head turning) using a commercial/conventional microswitch (e.g., a pressure device). A second group concerns studies that targeted a single nontypical (small) response (e.g., chin movements) using an experimental microswitch (e.g., an optic sensor). A third group concerns studies that targeted two or more responses (typical and nontypical) using combinations of commercial and experimental microswitches. A fourth group of studies, which is only briefly mentioned, involves combinations of responses employing microswitches and speech-generating devices (SGDs). The reason for the brief consideration of this last group is that the use of SGDs represents the topic of the next chapter of this book. The final part of this chapter analyzes the outcomes of the studies reviewed and their implications for daily programs and suggests questions for new research in the area.

Introduction

Microswitches are a main form of assistive technology developed to allow persons with extensive motor and multiple disabilities to activate environmental stimulus sources with small/simple responses (Holburn et al. 2004; Lancioni et al. 2001a, b, 2004a, b, c, 2008b; Mechling 2006). For example, a pressure microswitch (e.g., a touch pad) placed on the person's wheelchair tray could allow the person to activate brief periods of vibratory stimulation with a simple hand movement (rather than with the manipulation of the vibration device which would be impossible) (Lancioni et al. 2001a, 2008a, b). An optic microswitch (e.g., a mini photocell) fixed inside a box with objects could allow the person to obtain brief periods of musical stimulation by touching/moving the

G.E. Lancioni et al., *Assistive Technology: Interventions for Individuals with Severe/Profound and Multiple Disabilities*, Autism and Child Psychopathology Series, DOI 10.1007/978-1-4614-4229-5_2,

objects inside the box (Lancioni et al. 2002d, 2007b). A tilt microswitch arranged on the side of the person's head could allow the person to activate brief periods of visual stimulation with a simple head-turning or sideward head-tilting response (Lancioni et al. 2002b, 2008a, b). In practice, the microswitches may allow the persons to exercise control over environmental stimuli even when their motor (general) disabilities are so severe that they cannot manage any direct contact with and manipulation of those stimuli (Holburn et al. 2004; Lancioni et al. 2008b; Mechling 2006).

Without the availability of microswitches, those persons would need to rely on forms of environmental enrichment and stimulation handled by staff and families. These strategies could be useful to provide the persons an adequate input but (a) would emphasize their position/status of recipients of external initiative rather than of active agents who pursue the input on their own purpose (self-determination) and (b) would not really motivate them to develop any specific response schemes (i.e., any response that could be instrumental for them to access environmental stimulation). This lack of response development (learning) may be seen as a critically negative perspective with an impoverished social appearance of the persons and a seriously compromised outlook for their quality of life (Glickman et al. 1996; Lancioni et al. 2001a, b, c, d, 2007b, c, 2008a, b; Lachapelle et al. 2005; Mechling 2006; McDougall et al. 2010; Petry et al. 2009; Schalock et al. 2003).

A successful use of microswitches within habilitation programs for persons with profound and multiple disabilities would require at least three basic conditions to be met. First, a response should be identified that is already available in the person's repertoire (although at low frequencies) and is apparently easy (i.e., not excessively demanding and tiring) for the person to perform (Lancioni et al. 2002b, 2004c, 2008b). Second, a microswitch should be available (or possible to realize) that matches the response selected and can monitor it in a reliable manner and work as a dependable interface between the person's response and selected environmental events (i.e., forms of stimulation) (Lancioni et al. 2008b). Third, forms of stimulation should be identified that are apparently enjoyable for (preferred by) the person and thus motivating for him or her to (a) increase his or her responding to access them through the microswitch mediation and (b) maintain his or her responding levels over time (Crawford and Schuster 1993; Lancioni et al. 2008b).

This chapter provides an overview of studies using microswitches with persons with severe/profound and multiple disabilities. The studies are analyzed in terms of the responses the participants used, the microswitches adopted for those responses, the environmental events (stimulation) available in relation to the responses, and the general outcome. For practical (presentation) reasons, the studies are divided into several groups based on the responses targeted and the microswitches employed. A first group concerns studies that targeted a single typical response (e.g., head turning) using a commercial/conventional microswitch (e.g., a pressure device). A second group concerns studies that targeted a single nontypical (small) response (e.g., chin movements) using an experimental microswitch (e.g., an optic sensor). A third group concerns studies that targeted two or more responses (typical and nontypical) using combinations of commercial and experimental microswitches. A fourth group of studies, which is only briefly mentioned, involves combinations of responses employing microswitches and speech-generating devices (SGDs) (Lancioni et al. 2007a; Schlosser and Sigafoos 2006; Sigafoos et al. 2009). The reason for the brief consideration of this last group is that the use of SGDs is considered in depth in the next chapter of the book. The final part of this chapter analyzes the outcomes of the studies reviewed and their implications for daily programs and suggests questions for new research in the area. This chapter does not cover (a) the use of microswitches in combination with support devices to promote ambulation and (b) the use of microswitch clusters to reduce problem postures and behaviors while promoting adaptive responding, because these two topics will be analyzed in subsequent chapters of the book (Lancioni et al. 2005b, 2009c).

Studies Targeting a Single (Typical) Response with a Commercial/Conventional Microswitch

The most common responses used within this group of studies concerned head turning and hand pushing or variations of it (Leatherby et al. 1992; Saunders et al. 2003). The microswitches employed to monitor those responses generally consisted of pressure devices. Table 2.1 lists 10 studies belonging to this group (Dewson and Whiteley 1987; Gutowski 1996; Holburn et al. 2004; Lancioni et al. 2002c; Leatherby et al. 1992; Mechling 2006; Realon et al. 1988; Sandler and McLain 1987; Saunders et al. 2003; Wacker et al. 1988).

For example, Sandler and McLain (1987) conducted their investigation with five children between 6.5 and 8 years of age. Children were considered to be within the severe intellectual disability range, presented with extensive motor impairment, and used wheelchairs. One child was reported to be blind and another was diagnosed with hearing impairment. The study included five phases. Within each phase, the

Table 2.1 Studies targeting a single (typical) response with a commercial/conventional microswitch

Studies	Participants	Age (years)	Response types
Dewson and Whiteley (1987)	9	11–29	Head turning (pushing)
Sandler and McLain (1987)	5	6–8	Hand pushing
Realon et al. (1988)[a]	10	16–20	Hand, wrist, or elbow pushing
Wacker et al. (1988)[a]	5	16–20	Arm raising or hand pushing
Leatherby et al. (1992)[a]	5	7–13	Hand/arm pushing or pulling
Gutowski (1996)	2	39, 46	Hand pushing/closing
Lancioni et al. (2002c)	2	7, 14	Hand tapping
Saunders et al. (2003)	3	25–31	Head turning/pushing and hand/arm pushing
Holburn et al. (2004)	5	23–40	Head turning/pushing and hand, wrist, or fingers pushing
Mechling (2006)	3	6–19	Head turning and hand/arm movements

[a]The data refer to the first experiment reported in the study

children obtained a different type of stimulation contingent on their microswitch responding. Microswitches were pressure devices that were fitted to the wheelchair tray (during the four phases of the study in which food, praise, visual stimulation, and auditory stimulation were used contingent on the responses) or to a tray fixed to the arms of a small chair (during the phase of the study in which vestibular stimulation was applied). Food consequences consisted of a bite of a favorite edible, praise consisted of two positive statements, auditory and visual stimulation consisted of 10 s of music or 10 s of multicolor light input, and vestibular stimulation consisted of 10 s of gentle swinging. Participants seemed to have the highest (or very high) levels of responding during the vestibular stimulation condition. Lower levels of responding generally occurred during food or praise stimulation conditions.

Wacker et al. (1988) described a study with five participants between 13 and 20 years of age who were estimated to be functioning below the 1-year level. Four of them were provided with a contact/pressure microswitch, which was placed in front of them and could be activated with a simple hand-pressure response. The fifth participant was provided with a tilt microswitch combined with an arm-lifting response. When a participant activated the microswitch, one of the two toys available was activated for as long as the response lasted (i.e., for as long as the microswitch remained activated). The toys were changed across sessions according to an alternating treatment design. During the intervention condition, all participants increased the duration of their responding and also showed a preference for one of the toys over the other.

Gutowski (1996) employed pressure microswitches with two adults of 39 and 46 years of age. The microswitches were fixed on the wheelchair's armrest and in the participant's hands, respectively. The participants' microswitch activation through simple hand-pressure responses allowed them to access preferred environmental stimulation (i.e., small beverage quantities and brief music segments). Data indicated that both participants were able to increase their responding levels during the intervention period. This pointed out that the stimulation was motivating for them and the response-microswitch combination could be successfully used to access it.

Lancioni et al. (2002c) investigated the opportunity of using simple hand-tapping responses (spatially free and slightly forceful forms of contact with the tabletop) together with a vibration microswitch. The participants were two girls of 7 and 14 years of age who presented with intellectual, motor, and sensory disabilities and were in a wheelchair. Their hand-tapping responses activated the vibration microswitch and led to brief periods (below 10 s) of preferred stimulation including music, lights, and vibratory input. The responding level of both participants was fairly low during baseline conditions and increased in a decisive manner during the intervention periods indicating that it was sensitive to the stimulation that occurred contingent on it.

Holburn et al. (2004) carried out a study with five participants between 23 and 40 years of age who had a diagnosis of profound intellectual disability and extensive motor impairment requiring the use of wheelchairs. The participants did not have any functional communication system and depended on caregivers for their daily needs as well as stimulation input. The microswitches consisted of pressure devices that could be activated with hand or head movements. The stimuli that the participants received contingent on their responses consisted of visual images presented on a computer screen, which could be supplemented by sound effects. A series of 50 images were available within each session. The results indicated that response increases were substantial in two participants, moderate in a third participant, and vague/limited in the final two participants.

Mechling (2006) taught three participants to use hand/arm movements and head-turning responses in combination with pressure microswitches to access various environmental stimuli. The participants were between 6 and 19 years of age and presented with profound intellectual disabilities and serious motor impairment. The study included nine sessions of 9 min. Every session contained three intervention sections of 3 min. Each section involved a specific stimulus condition, that is, a specific type of consequence occurring contingent on the responses per 10 s at each response. The stimulus conditions involved adapted toys and devices, commercial cause-and-effect software, and instructor-created video programs. Subsequent to this period aimed at verifying possible differences in responding under the different stimulus condition, a program supplement was implemented. Such a supplement consisted of three sessions, in which only the stimulus condition that had promoted the highest level of responding was used. The results of the first assessment period showed that the level of responding was highest (i.e., between five and nine responses per section) with the instructor-created video programs. During the program supplement, the response level remained satisfactory for all three participants.

Studies Targeting a Single (Nontypical) Response with a New/Experimental Microswitch

The typical responses and commercial microswitches examined above, albeit apparently simple and immediate, may not suit a number of persons with pervasive disabilities and a minimal behavioral (motor) repertoire (Lancioni et al. 2005c, 2008b). With regard to those persons, the professional is left with two options: (a) excluding them from participation in microswitch programs or (b) resorting to the use of small, nontypical responses that might be more feasible for them and to the development of new microswitch devices that can detect such responses. Those responses could include vocalization (voice emissions), eyelid or chin movements, and minimal hand closures or finger movements (Lancioni et al. 2006f, 2009b). Table 2.2 provides a list of studies, in each of which new/experimental microswitch technology was used for monitoring a single, nontypical response. The responses covered by the studies were *vocalization* (Lancioni et al. 2001c, 2005d, 2008a), *chin and mouth/lip movements* (Lancioni et al. 2004a, c, 2006c, 2010c, 2011), *eyelid movements* (Lancioni et al. 2005a, 2006f, 2009a, b), *forehead or eyebrow movements* (Lancioni et al. 2007b, 2009a, 2011), and *hand closure* (Lancioni et al. 2007c, 2009b, c).

Table 2.2 Studies targeting a single (nontypical) response with a new/experimental microswitch

Studies	Participants	Age (years)	Response types
Lancioni et al. (2001c)	2	7, 10	Vocalization
Lancioni et al. (2005d)	1	8	Vocalization
Lancioni et al. (2008a)	1	22	Vocalization
Lancioni et al. (2004a)	1	18	Chin movements
Lancioni et al. (2004c)	1	6	Chin movements
Lancioni et al. (2006c)	2	7.5, 8	Chin movements
Lancioni et al. (2010c)	1	41	Lip movements
Lancioni et al. (2011)	1	5.5	Partial mouth closing
Lancioni et al. (2005a)	1	9	Eyelid movements
Lancioni et al. (2006f)	2	10, 12	Eyelid movements
Lancioni et al. (2009a)	1	36	Eyelid movements
Lancioni et al. (2009b)	1	26	Eyelid movements
Lancioni et al. (2007b)	2	6, 14	Forehead skin movements
Lancioni et al. (2009a)	1	68	Eyebrow movements
Lancioni et al. (2011)	1	7.5	Eyebrow movements
Lancioni et al. (2007c)	2	5, 21	Hand closure
Lancioni et al. (2009a)	1	68	Hand closure
Lancioni et al. (2009d)	1	65	Hand closure

Vocalization

The first study targeting this response (Lancioni et al. 2001c) was carried out with two participants of 7 and 10 years of age. Both had pervasive multiple disabilities with minimal motor repertoires, but displayed spontaneous vocal emissions. These emissions were considered a relevant resource and targeted through a new (specifically built) microswitch. The new microswitch consisted of a battery-powered, sound-detecting device connected to a throat microphone (not affected by environmental noise), which was held at the participants' larynx, with a simple neckband (see Fig. 2.1). During the intervention phase, vocalization responses activated the microswitch, which in turn led to the occurrence of brief periods of preferred stimulation. The stimulation was regulated through an electronic control system, which was connected to the microswitch and the stimulation source. Data showed that during that phase, the participants' level of vocalization responses increased substantially over the baseline and remained consistent suggesting that (a) an association between responses and stimulation had occurred and (b) stimulation had (and maintained) motivating/reinforcing effects.

The aforementioned technology was upgraded in a study by Lancioni et al. (2005d), which involved a girl of 8 years of age with profound multiple disabilities. The upgrading was decided because the use of a contact (throat) microswitch alone can result in false activations if the person has heavily congested tracheal areas, drops his or her head forward, or presents dystonic head movements. The upgrading aimed at limiting these potential drawbacks consisted of the introduction of an

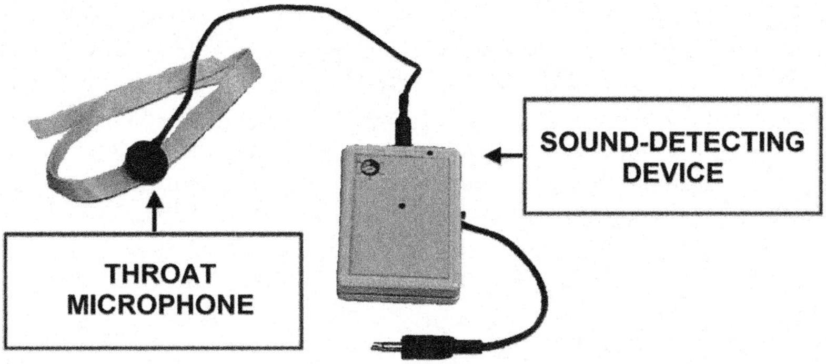

Fig. 2.1 Pictorial representation of the battery-powered, sound-detecting device connected to the throat microphone

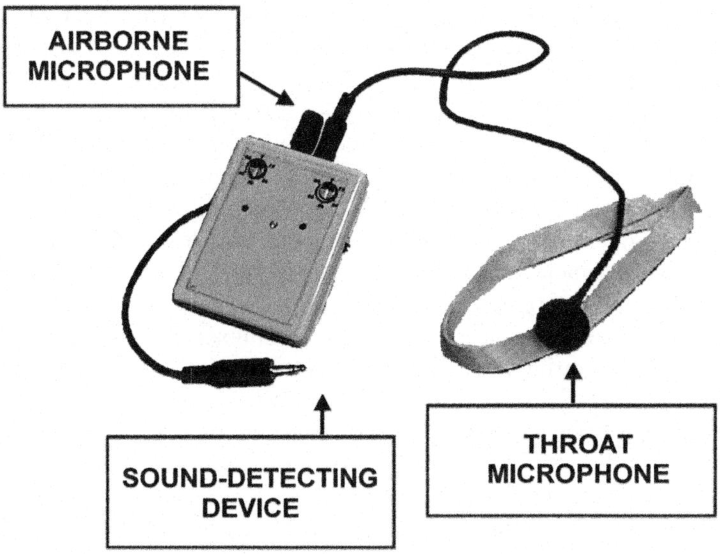

Fig. 2.2 Pictorial representation of the battery-powered, sound-detecting device connected to the throat microphone and an airborne microphone

airborne microphone parallel to the throat microphone (see Fig. 2.2). Activation of the microswitch (and stimulation) would occur only if both microphones were triggered. The girl's responding increased. The solution seemed adequate to eliminate false activations that could previously occur in absence of vocal emissions.

Lancioni et al. (2008a) estimated the levels of false microswitch activations using a vocalization microswitch with the throat microphone only and a vocalization microswitch with the combination of throat and the airborne microphones. The participant was a man of 22 years of age who had congenital encephalopathy with profound intellectual disability, spastic tetraparesis, and minimal residual vision. During the 46 intervention sessions involving the microswitch with throat microphone only, the participant had a mean of over 40 responses per session with over 6 responses per session being rated as false-positives. During the 48 intervention sessions involving the microswitch with both microphones, the mean frequency of responses per session was largely similar, but the frequency of responses rated as false-positives was below one per session.

Chin and Mouth/Lip Movements

Several studies have been carried out using chin and mouth/lip movements as response. For example, Lancioni et al. (2006c) conducted two single-case studies including a 7.5-year-old girl and an 8-year-old boy, respectively. The children were reported to be functioning in the severe or profound intellectual disability range with minimal residual vision or blindness, to have pervasive motor disabilities without apparently useful response schemes, and to lack any practical interaction with their surroundings. The response selected for them as a plausible (reliable) motor expression to control environmental events was a downward chin movement. The microswitch developed to monitor the response with the girl consisted of (a) a position sensor hidden inside a box which was fixed to the side of a hat, (b) an electronic regulation unit, and (c) a light band, which was tied to the position sensor and to the other side of the hat, and passed under the girl's chin (see Fig. 2.3). When the girl produced a downward movement of the chin, pulling the band and thus the position sensor, the regulation unit sent a signal to an electronic control unit, which (during intervention) turned on preferred stimuli for brief periods of time.

The microswitch developed for the boy was different, as he did not like the band touching his face. It involved a hat that supported a light structure passing in front of his face (without touching any part of it) and ending immediately below his chin. The end of this structure contained an optic sensor, which was activated as soon as the chin approached it (i.e., as soon as a downward movement of the chin occurred) (see Fig. 2.4). When the optic sensor was activated, the regulation unit sent a signal to an electronic control system, and this led to brief stimulation periods (i.e., during the intervention). The outcomes of the studies with the two microswitches (and the two children) were highly satisfactory. Both children learned to use the microswitches rapidly and increased their level of responding and access to stimulation.

A response characterized by movements of the lips (which could also encompass chin and jaw movements and thus resemble the one mentioned above) was recently targeted with a 41-year-old woman who had suffered severe brain injury and coma following a car accident (Lancioni et al. 2010c). She had a diagnosis of minimally conscious state and presented with pervasive neuromotor disabilities resulting in a

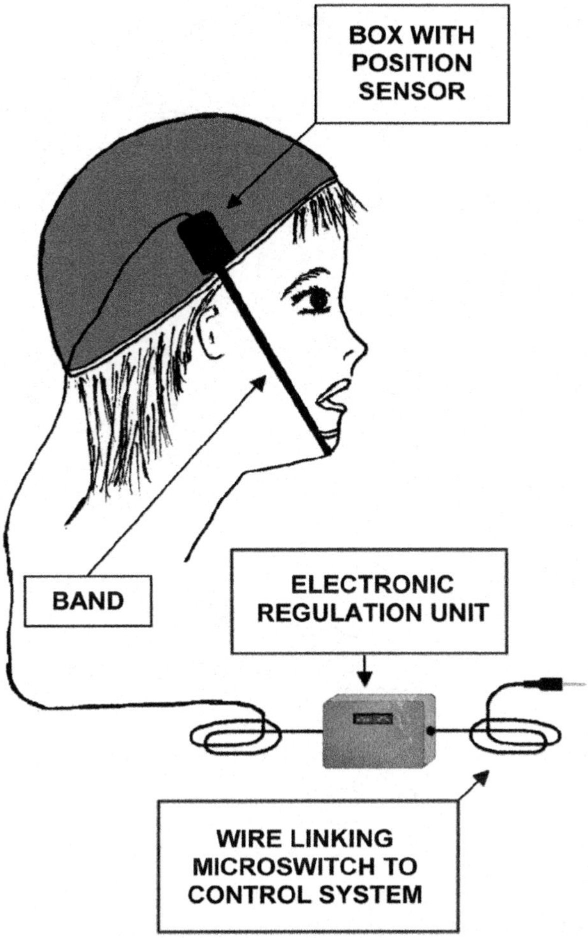

Fig. 2.3 Schematic representation of the box with the position sensor, the band tied to the position sensor and to the other side of the hat the child wore, and the electronic regulation unit

totally static position. A variation of the aforementioned forms of microswitch was developed to detect the response. It included two optic sensors consisting of an infrared light-emitting diode and a mini infrared light-detection unit. The sensors were attached to a metal support fixed to the woman's chin. The aforementioned sensors were normally directed at the upper lip and at the mouth cavity, respectively (see Fig. 2.5, Frame 1) (i.e., as the woman rested static with her mouth semi-open and lips apart). When the woman's lips moved closer together or further apart, the fixation point(s) of the sensors changed (see Fig. 2.5, Frames 2 and 3) and produced microswitch activations. Those activations (i.e., through an electronic control system) led to the occurrence of brief periods of preferred stimulation during the intervention phases. The woman showed clear increases in the frequency of her lip movements during those phases as compared to baseline periods.

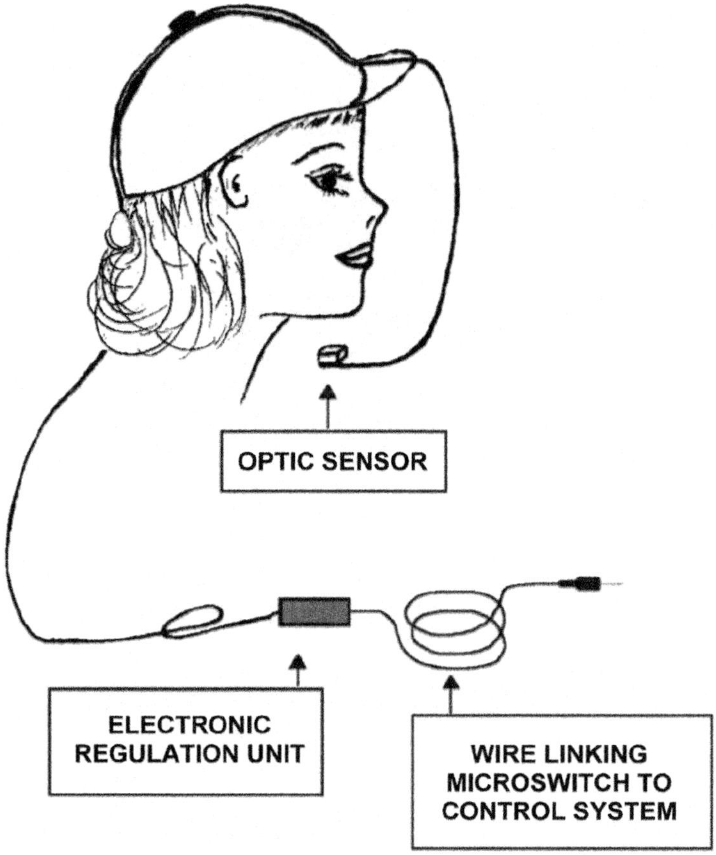

Fig. 2.4 Schematic representation of the optic sensor held under the child's chin and of the electronic regulation unit

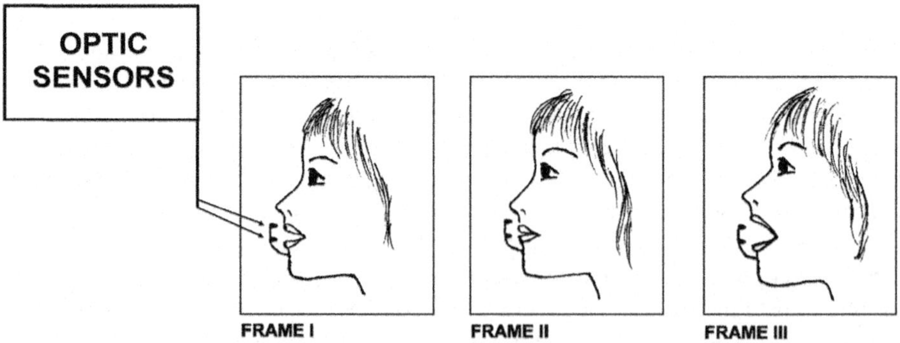

Fig. 2.5 Schematic representation of optic sensors used for monitoring the woman's regular lip position (Frame 1) and two possible lip-position changes (Frames 2 and 3)

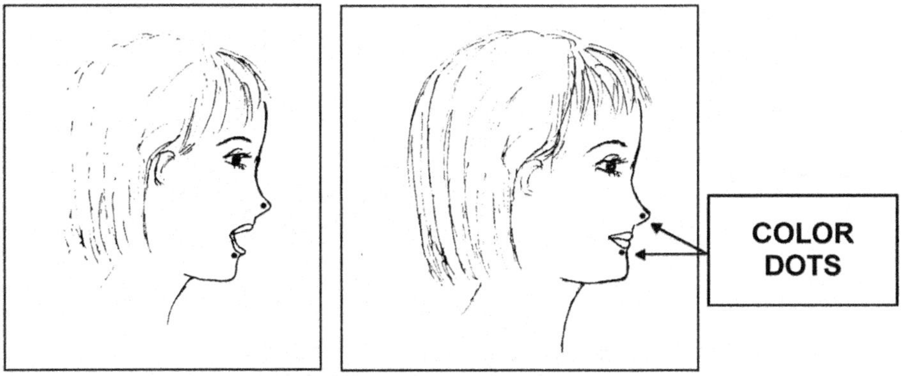

Fig. 2.6 Schematic representation of possible color dots used to detect mouth closing with a camera-based microswitch

Lancioni et al. (2011) targeted a partial mouth-closing response in a child with multiple disabilities using a camera-based microswitch. The child was nearly 5.5 years old and had a diagnosis of congenital encephalopathy linked to a polymalformative syndrome with spastic tetraparesis, minimal residual vision, and other neurophysiological disabilities. The response was monitored through a camera connected to a computer system provided with specific software. The camera was positioned at about 1 m from the child's face, in which two small color dots were drawn to allow the camera and computer to detect the response. The dots were on the child's nose and under her lower lip (see Fig. 2.6). When the distance between the barycenter of the two dots showed a reduction of over 25 % of its original (reference) value, the computer recorded a mouth-closing response. This in turn led to brief stimulation events throughout the intervention. The child's response frequency increased largely as a consequence of the intervention conditions.

Eyelid Movements

Studies have assessed the two main aspects of the response, that is, eyelid closure and eyelid lifting. Regarding eyelid closure, response recording could focus on a single blink or repeated blinks. An early study by Lancioni et al. (2005a) examined the possibility of using a repeated-blink response with a boy of 9 years of age with profound multiple disabilities and minimal motor behavior. The response, which was to include two blinks within a 2-s interval, was already present in the child's repertoire but at a relatively low frequency. The microswitch for the response included (a) an optic sensor mounted on an eyeglasses frame that the boy wore during the sessions and (b) a regulation unit and a control system that produced and registered a response signal, respectively, when the child performed two blinks within a 2-s interval (see Fig. 2.7). Response performance allowed access to brief

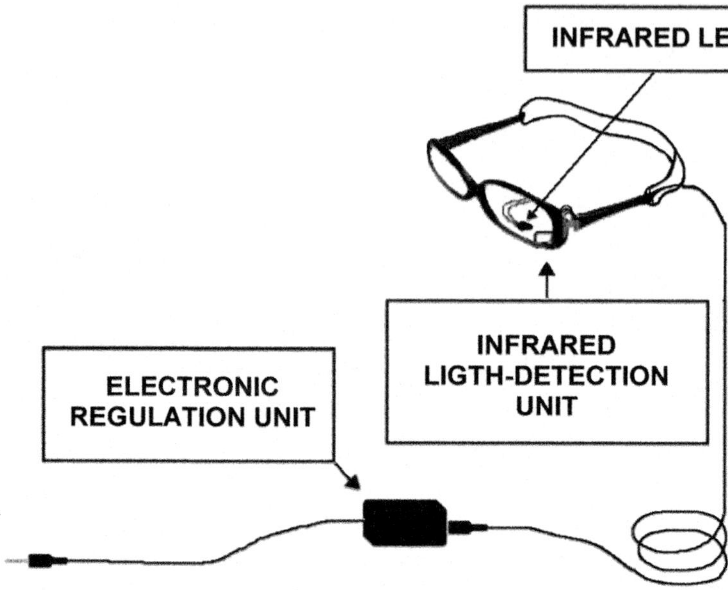

Fig. 2.7 Schematic representation of an optic sensor (infrared LED and infrared light-detection unit) mounted on an eyeglasses frame and connected to an electronic regulation unit

periods of preferred stimulation during the intervention periods. Data showed that the child's response rates had a clear increase during those periods compared to the baseline phases.

Lancioni et al. (2006f) extended the early research with the use of eyelid movements with two children of 10 and 12 years of age. The response selected for these children was not a repeated blink (as in the aforementioned study), but an upward eyelid movement, that is, an eyelid lifting. This consisted of raising one eyelid or both eyelids, as it would occur when looking at an object placed in an elevated position relative to the person. This response, which was considered more suitable for these children, was monitored with an adapted version of the microswitch technology described above. Specifically, the optic sensors mounted on eyeglasses frames were not to detect the eyelid closures (i.e., the transition from the eye pupil to the eyelid, that is, from a dark to a light component of the eye) but the eyelid lifting (i.e., the transition from the eyelid to the eye pupil). The performance of the target response allowed the participants to access brief periods of preferred visual, auditory, and vibrotactile stimulation. Data showed that both children were able to learn to use the response successfully. In other words, they displayed increased frequencies of the response during the intervention (i.e., when stimulation was available contingent on it) as opposed to the baseline condition (i.e., when stimulation was not available).

The requirement of targeting double blinking or upward eyelid movements as specific responses may be unavoidable when the participants display relatively (and consistently) high frequencies of eye-blinking responses. Whenever the participant displays relatively low blinking frequencies, however, a single-blink response might be considered as a viable option. In line with this notion, Lancioni et al. (2009a, b) reported two applications of the single-blink response. The first application concerned a woman of 36 years of age who had suffered severe brain injury and coma subsequent to a road accident. The woman had a diagnosis of vegetative state and was exposed to a learning assessment procedure. The optic microswitch used to monitor the response was fixed on the woman's forehead. Activation of the microswitch triggered an electronic control system that, in turn, started brief occasions of auditory and/or visual stimulation. Data showed relatively low (or declining) response frequencies during the baseline phases, increased responding during the intervention phases, and partial response declines during a control condition (i.e., noncontingent stimulation). These data were thought to show signs of a nonreflective minimal level of consciousness and consequently prompt a change of diagnosis for the participant.

The second application of the single-blink response concerned a man of 26 years of age who had suffered severe brain injury and coma subsequent to a road accident. At the time of the study, he had a diagnosis of minimally conscious state with pervasive neuromotor disabilities. The microswitch used with him was an adapted version of the optic sensor described above (Lancioni et al. 2005a, 2006f). The performance of each single-blink response was followed by a brief access to preferred stimulation during the intervention phases. Data showed that the response frequency during those phases increased significantly and remained high.

Forehead and Eyebrow Movements

Lancioni et al. (2007b) assessed the feasibility of using small upward or downward movements of the forehead skin as a response for two participants with profound multiple disabilities of 6 and 14 years of age. The microswitch used to monitor such a response consisted of an optic sensor (barcode reader) with an electronic regulation unit and a small tag with horizontal bars. The tag was pasted on the participants' forehead, and the optic sensor was held in front of the tag via a light support structure (see Fig. 2.8). During the intervention, small movements of the tag (occurring in concomitance with small upward or downward movements of the forehead skin) triggered the microswitch system. This activated a control system that ensured brief periods of preferred stimulation. Both participants had a clear response increase during the intervention phases of the study.

Lancioni et al. (2009a) investigated the use of eyebrow lifting as the target response with a man of 68 years of age. The man had suffered traumatic brain injury and coma and had a diagnosis of minimally conscious state and pervasive neuromotor disabilities at the time of the study. The microswitch adopted for this response was a modified version of the optic sensor used in the studies targeting eyelid closures and eyelid upward movements (see above). The microswitch was fixed on the man's forehead (see Fig. 2.9). During the intervention phases of the study, eyebrow lifting resulting in microswitch activation allowed the man brief access to preferred visual stimuli (i.e., video clips of favorite events). Data showed that his response frequency increased largely during those phases as compared to the baseline.

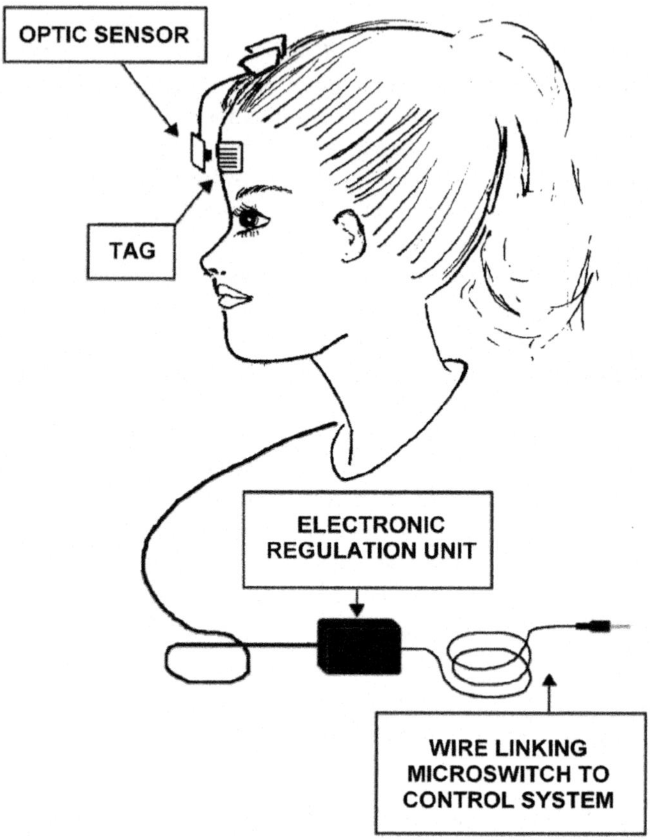

Fig. 2.8 Schematic representation of an optic sensor (barcode reader), a small tag with horizontal bars, and an electronic regulation unit used to detect forehead skin movements

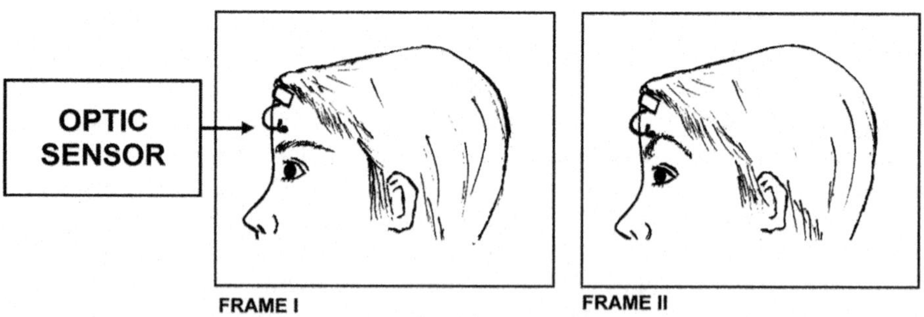

Fig. 2.9 Schematic representation of an optic sensor used for pointing to the forehead (Frame 1) and to the eyebrow (Frame 2)

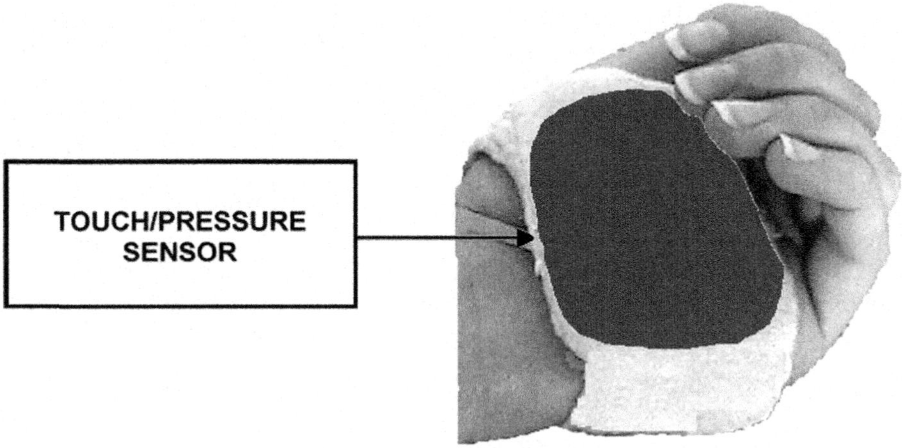

Fig. 2.10 Schematic representation of a touch/pressure sensor fixed to the person's hand

A recent study (Lancioni et al. 2011) targeted the aforementioned eyebrow-lifting response with the use of a camera-based microswitch, such as that described above for mouth closing. The participant was a boy of about 7.5 years of age who had suffered severe brain hemorrhage at 1 year of age with consequent development of spastic tetraparesis, total blindness, and epilepsy as well as profound intellectual disability and lack of self-help and communication skills. The boy was provided with two small color dots above the right eyebrow and on the top right side of the forehead. The camera and computer detected a response when the distance between the barycenters of the dots decreased of about 12 %. Response frequencies increased during the intervention, that is, when they were followed by brief (preferred) stimulation events.

Hand Closure

Lancioni et al. (2007c) reported the use of small hand-closure movements as the response with two participants of 5 and 21 years of age. The response, which seemed highly suitable (relatively easy) for persons who tend to have their hands partially closed, consisted of the participants' fingers touching or pressing on a microswitch fixed to the palm of their hand. The microswitch involved a two-membrane thin device. The external membrane (i.e., the one exposed to direct contact with the participants' fingers) was a touch-sensitive sensor and was thus activated by light contact with the fingers. The internal membrane was a pressure sensor that would be activated if the participants applied a pressure/weight of about 20 g on it (see Fig. 2.10). During the intervention, the response allowed the participants to access brief periods of stimulation including combinations of preferred visual, auditory, and vibrotactile events. Data showed that both participants increased their response frequency (use of the microswitch) as a consequence of the intervention conditions.

Lancioni et al. (2009a, d) reported an additional use of the hand-closure response and the two-membrane microswitch for two post-coma adults with a diagnosis of vegetative state. The two participants who were 68 and 65 years old were exposed to a learning assessment procedure in which each hand-closure response was followed by a brief stimulation period. The response had a relatively low (or declining) frequency during the baseline phases, increased during the intervention phases, and declined to an intermediate level (i.e., between baseline and intervention) during a control condition. These results were taken to suggest that the participants had a nonreflective minimal level of consciousness.

Studies Targeting Two or More Responses with Experimental and Commercial Microswitches

The acquisition of a specific response with a microswitch may be considered a critical step to enable persons with pervasive and multiple disabilities to establish a form of relation with the outside world and manage control of stimulation events. For many of these persons, acquiring the use of one response and one microswitch may be only a transitory stage in their educational program. In particular, they might have the ability to acquire more responses with other microswitches with obvious benefits in terms of activity, stimulation input, and possibly choice. Indeed, the use of multiple responses/microswitches would allow the participant to extend and vary his or her behavioral engagement, enrich and diversify his or her stimulation opportunities, and eventually choose between the different stimuli available, based on preferences and other practical conditions. Table 2.3 provides a list of eight studies

Table 2.3 Studies targeting two or more responses with experimental and commercial microswitches

Studies	Participants	Age (years)	Response types
Sullivan et al. (1995)	1	3.5	Two responses: head and hand movements
Lancioni et al. (2002a)	2	8, 12	Three responses per participant: vocalization, head, and hand movements
Lancioni et al. (2003)	1	16.5	Two responses: hand to forehead and knee shaking
Lancioni et al. (2004b)	2	26, 27	Three or four responses per participant: feet and leg movements
Lancioni et al. (2006b)	3	7–16	Two responses per participant: vocalization and chin, mouth, knee, and hand movements
Lancioni et al. (2009b)	1	45	Two responses: head and foot movements
Lancioni et al. (2010b)	2	53, 56	Two responses per participant: finger, hand, eyelid, and head movements
Lancioni et al. (2010d)	2	79, 52	Two responses per participant: right and left head turning or bending

assessing the combined use of two or more microswitches (Lancioni et al. 2002a, 2003, 2004b, 2006b, 2009b, 2010b, d; Sullivan et al. 1995).

Sullivan et al. (1995) reported an early research study aimed at targeting two responses with two separate microswitches. The authors worked with a girl who was 3.5 years of age and had a diagnosis of Rett syndrome. The two responses targeted with her consisted of head backward movements and hand-pushing/stroking movements. These responses were monitored through the use of commercially available pressure microswitches. The microswitches were simultaneously available, and the girl could activate either one of them obtaining access to different types of preferred stimuli (e.g., musical toys and tapes). The results showed that the girl increased the frequency of both responses as a consequence of the intervention conditions.

Lancioni et al. (2002a) reported a study in which two children of 8 and 12 years of age were involved. The three responses targeted for each participant concerned vocalization, hand movements (pushing/stroking), and head movements. Each response allowed access to a specific set of stimuli during the intervention phases in which it was involved. The study started with baseline on each of the responses, and then intervention focused on the first one of them. When the participants showed a clear increase of this response, a new baseline was carried out on the second response. Thereafter, intervention started on it. Increases of this second response led to an intervention period in which both responses and microswitches were available within each session. That is, the participant could carry out any of them and receive the stimulation related to it. Once the participant had shown successful performance with these two responses/microswitches, a final baseline was carried out on the third response/microswitch. This was followed by intervention on this last combination and then intervention on all three responses and microswitches. At the last stage of the program, the participant could perform any of the responses using the related microswitch and accessing specific stimuli. This response freedom ensured an extensive and differentiated engagement and an important opportunity to choose among three sets of preferred stimuli. Data indicated that both participants succeeded in acquiring the responses and had an increased and consistent use of all three of them.

Lancioni et al. (2003) worked with an adolescent who presented with microcephaly, spastic tetraparesis, severe scoliosis, and blindness. She was classified as functioning in the profound intellectual disability range, had no speech or other forms of communication, and was fitted with a feeding tube. The two responses selected for the study consisted of bringing the hand to the forehead and shaking the knee. The microswitch used for the first response consisted of twin optic sensors fixed to a headband that the participant wore. The microswitch for knee shaking consisted of a tilt-like device. After the initial baseline on both responses, the intervention focused on the first response. The emission of the response led to brief periods of visual and auditory stimulation. Once this response increased, a new baseline and intervention occurred on the second response. The emission of this response during the intervention led to brief stimulation including also vibratory input. Data showed that the participant increased the frequency of each response as a consequence of the intervention conditions.

Lancioni et al. (2004b) targeted simple foot and leg movements of two adults (wheelchair users) as responses to enhance through a microswitch-based intervention. The two participants were 26 and 27 years old, were classified as functioning in the profound intellectual disability range, were totally blind, and did not possess self-help skills. They needed a wheelchair due to spasticity, scoliosis, and hip or foot abnormalities. The responses selected for the first participant consisted of pulling up the front part of his feet together and raising the left or the right leg. The microswitch for the first response was a pressure device, which was released by the response. The microswitches for the leg responses were tilt devices. The responses selected for the second participant consisted of raising the right leg or the left leg and pushing down with the left or the right foot. The microswitches for the leg responses were tilt devices. The microswitches for the foot responses were pressure devices. The first participant started with a baseline on all responses, and then the intervention focused on feet pulling. The occurrence of the response produced brief periods of stimulation (e.g., music or vibratory stimulation). Increased frequencies on this response led to a new baseline on the other two responses and then intervention on them, in succession. The second participant started with baseline on all responses, which led to intervention on the leg responses. Increased frequencies on these responses led to focus the intervention on the foot responses. Again, intervention ensured that brief periods of preferred stimulation followed the emission of the responses. Results indicated that both participants were highly successful in increasing all the responses targeted.

Lancioni et al. (2006b) carried out a study with three participants and targeted two responses for each of them. The participants were between 7 and 16 years of age and presented with severe/profound intellectual disabilities and extensive motor impairment. The responses were vocalization and repeated chin movements, light knee movement and minimal movement of a grid, and mouth closing and hand opening for the three participants, respectively. The microswitches employed for vocalization and chin movements matched those previously described for the same responses (Lancioni et al. 2001c, 2006c). The microswitches employed for mouth closing and hand opening consisted of specially adapted versions of the initial microswitch developed for chin movements (Lancioni et al. 2006c). The microswitches employed for knee and grid movements were combinations of tilt devices. Each participant started with baseline on the two responses. Then intervention on these responses and related microswitches was carried out sequentially. Once the second response had been consolidated, the intervention involved both responses (i.e., both microswitches were simultaneously available during the sessions and the participant received specific stimulation events for each response). In essence, the participants could choose between responses/microswitches and, more importantly, between the stimuli linked to them. Eventually, the study assessed the participants' preferences. That is, it determined whether the participants' preference for one response or the other was to be ascribed to the stimuli following that response (i.e., to the higher motivational power of those stimuli) or was also due to a preference for the response as such. Data showed that all three participants acquired the two responses selected for them. They also displayed obvious differences in the frequencies of the responses. An analysis of those differences suggested that they (a) were related to the stimuli following the responses for two of the participants and (b) were partially related to the impact of the stimuli and partially due to the characteristics/suitability of the responses for the third participant.

Lancioni et al. (2009b) carried out a study with a man of 45 years of age who had suffered extensive brain injury and coma following cerebral aneurism rupture. At the time of the study, the man was diagnosed with a minimally conscious state and extensive neuromotor disabilities. The responses targeted for him were head and foot movements. The microswitches adopted for these responses consisted of pressure devices, which were fixed at the wheelchair's headrest, and a combination of tilt and pressure devices, which were linked to the man's right foot. The responses (and microswitches) were exposed to intervention conditions in sequence and then targeted simultaneously throughout the sessions. During intervention, the head-movement response (activating the headrest's pressure devices) turned on short video clips; the foot-movement response (activating the combination of sensors on it) turned on brief audio recordings. The man learned to use both responses and related microswitches through the intervention phases. He also continued to have high responding levels during the later stages of the study, that is, when both microswitches were available simultaneously within the sessions. Apparently, he had a preference for the foot-movement response.

Lancioni et al. (2010d) worked with two post-coma adults (a woman and a man) of 79 and 52 years of age, who presented with a minimally conscious state and extensive neuromotor disabilities. The responses targeted for the first participant were right and left head turning. The responses targeted for the second participant consisted of right and left head bending. The microswitches used for the head-turning responses were tilt devices fixed on a headband that the participant (who was lying in bed) wore during the sessions. The microswitches used for the head-bending responses consisted of optic microswitches fixed on the participant's shoulders (to avoid any contact with his face and head). During the intervention phases of the study, microswitch activation triggered a control system that in turn started brief periods of preferred stimulation. In particular, popular songs and prayers or religious choirs were available for the right and left head turning of the first participant, respectively. Film clips of popular stories and of natural scenes were used for the right and left head bending of the second participant, respectively. Initially, baseline assessment was carried out on both responses. Subsequently, intervention (with the occurrence of brief stimulation periods) focused on the first response. Once this response increased, a new baseline and intervention were carried out on the second response. Finally, intervention was extended to both responses, that is, the participants had the two microswitches available simultaneously and obtained specific stimulation events for each of the responses. Data showed that the participants increased their responding during the intervention phases, with an apparent preference for one of the responses and related stimulation (first participant) or no significant differences between responses (second participant).

Studies Targeting Two or More Responses with Microswitches and Speech-Generating Devices (SGDs)

The largely successful use of single and multiple microswitches, as reviewed above, provides encouraging evidence as to the potential and applicability of these technological resources within daily programs for persons with severe/profound and multiple disabilities. These resources, in fact, may represent a most immediate and valuable tool to enable the persons to pursue positive engagement, independent stimulation access, and choice. The use of these resources may be considered a critical component of any rehabilitation context for two main reasons. First, as suggested above, they can be instrumental to help the participants develop forms of activity and independence. Moreover, they are really essential to promote learning and consolidation of specific responses that extend the person's behavior repertoire and empower him or her (i.e., allow him or her to manage environmental events) (Holburn et al. 2004; Lancioni et al. 2008b). Second, they can be a valid and useful supplement to the direct intervention of rehabilitation and care staff. In no context, in fact, one can expect the presence of staff personnel to be uninterrupted and guarantee continuous educational input (Lancioni et al. 2008b).

Acknowledging the extremely important functions of microswitch technology may not totally eliminate a sense of caution about the use of such technology. The caution would originate from the realization that the aforementioned technology can promote the persons' access to (control of) a variety of environmental stimuli, but cannot help them satisfy any desires they might have about contact/interaction with their caregiver. Obviously, such need of caution would only be realistic and credible when the microswitch technology is used for relatively long sessions and/or a large number of sessions during the day. In those situations (and probably in less concerning ones as well), a reassuring approach might consist of supplementing conventional microswitch technology with an SGD or voice output communication aid (VOCA). The microswitch technology would ensure that the participant continues to access environmental stimuli independently. The SGD/VOCA would enable the participant to ask for caregiver contact whenever he or she desires to have such a contact. The use of SGD/VOCA technology will be the focus of the next chapter of this book. Only two studies combining the use of microswitch and SGD technology will be summarized here to illustrate the issue and the procedural conditions.

For example, Lancioni et al. (2008c) carried out a study, in which three responses were selected for each of the two participants who were 16 and 18 years old and presented with multiple (intellectual, sensory, and motor) disabilities. Two responses involved the use of microswitches and a one the use of an SGD/VOCA. The responses selected for the microswitches consisted of head and hand movements for both participants. The responses selected for the SGD consisted of vocalization for one participant and a specific hand movement for the other participant. Initially, the intervention focused on each of the two microswitches individually. When responding had increased, they were made available simultaneously and the participants could choose between them and the stimuli linked to them. Subsequently, the intervention focused on the SGD. Once responding to it had increased, the SGD and the two microswitches were made available simultaneously. At that point, the participants could choose among the three opportunities. Activation of the microswitches allowed them to access different sets of preferred stimuli (e.g., musical and visual items). Activation of the SGD triggered a vocal output apparatus, which emitted a verbal request of attention directed to the caregiver. The caregiver would respond to the requests either verbally or verbally and physically. Verbal responding consisted of presenting complimentary/support sentences and occurred for about two-thirds of the SGD requests. Verbal and physical responding consisted of talking to and touching/caressing or kissing the participant briefly and occurred for about one-third of the SGD requests. The use of the two different types of responding and their relative ratios was decided for practical reasons. Preponderance of verbal responding was thought to allow the caregiver to largely maintain his or her other/regular duties during the intervention program. The outcome of the study was positive for both participants. They learned to use the microswitches and the SGD. A majority of their responses (i.e., about three-fourths of them) concerned the use of microswitches.

Lancioni et al. (2009e) conducted a study with two post-coma persons of 35 and 60 years of age, who were diagnosed to be in a minimally conscious state and presented with extensive motor disabilities. After the initial baseline, the study involved an intervention period aimed at strengthening one of the two responses available together with a microswitch device. The microswitch consisted of a touch-sensitive device fixed onto the leg for one participant and of a touch- and pressure-sensitive device fixed into the palm of the hand for the other participant. Microswitch activation allowed them access to brief periods of preferred stimulation (e.g., music). Once they had learned to use the microswitch, the SGD was introduced. This consisted of (a) a wobble-like device attached to the stomach that could be activated by a general hand movement for one participant and (b) tilt devices attached to the foot that could be activated through slight foot movement for the other participant. Activation of the SGD produced a call for the caregiver. In response to the call, the caregiver talked to the participant and engaged him or her in watching or listening to a variety of stimuli. Once the participants had learned to use the SGD, the program involved the simultaneous availability of the microswitch and the SGD so that the participants could use any of them at will. The results showed that both participants were successful in acquiring the use of the microswitch and the SGD and increased their independent access to preferred stimulation and their interaction with the caregiver, favoring one or the other at different times.

Discussion

Outcome of the Studies

The positive results generally reported by the studies using microswitches underline the importance of adopting these forms of assistive technology for persons with severe/profound and multiple disabilities (Lancioni et al. 2008b, 2009a, b, c; Shih et al. 2010; Sigafoos et al. 2009). Obtaining a successful outcome in intervention programs such as those examined in this overview may require a number of conditions to be met. One of those conditions concerns the response difficulty/cost, which should not be too high for the participant. More specifically, the likelihood of success is greater if the response is in the person's repertoire and requires a fairly low level of effort to be performed (Lancioni et al. 2005c, 2008b, 2010d). A second condition concerns the availability of microswitches suitable for the responses. Small, nontypical responses may need new and experimental technical solutions. An array of those solutions has been presented in this chapter. Some of those solutions are quite simple and immediate. Others may be more difficult to realize and afford within daily contexts. A third condition concerns the stimulus events selected for the participant's response(s). These events should have a motivating (reinforcing) power, and their positive/reinforcing value for the participant should exceed the efforts required of him or her to perform the response(s) (Kazdin 2001). A fourth condition concerns the intervention length, which (a) would need to be adapted to the participant's learning characteristics and essentially (b) should be significantly extended with participants who have more severe (disadvantaged) conditions (Catania 2007; Kazdin 2001; Lancioni et al. 2001a, 2009a; Saunders et al. 2003).

The most immediate evidence of the positive outcomes of the studies reviewed was the participants' increased frequencies of responses. Other seemingly important pieces of evidence, which were recorded only in some of the study, could be (a) the indices of happiness or unhappiness of the participants and (b) the opinion of staff personnel, family members, or other raters about the technology and its application impact and overall effects (Dillon and Carr 2007; Lancioni et al. 2006d, e, 2007d, 2008b). With regard to the first point, for example, Lancioni et al. (2006d) assessed the mood of the three children involved in a microswitch-based study, in which each child could use a microswitch to access brief periods of preferred stimulation. The results indicated that two of the children had clear increases in indices of happiness during the intervention. The third child had a decrease (a virtual elimination) of indices of unhappiness (i.e., frowning and crying) during the intervention.

With regard to the second point, Lancioni et al. (2006a) conducted a social validation study in which 140 teacher trainees and 84 parents were involved in rating microswitch-based programs versus interaction or stimulation conditions for participants with multiple disabilities. All raters (teacher trainees and parents) scored the two conditions on a seven-item questionnaire concerning the participants' apparent enjoyment of the two conditions, the possible impact of those conditions, and the raters' own view on the likableness (acceptability) of those conditions. Data indicated that both groups of raters provided the microswitch programs with higher (more positive) scoring on all seven items. These scores seemed to constitute a very strong endorsement of the microswitch-based programs, which supplemented in a meaningful manner the positive outcomes of the programs in terms of participants' response frequencies.

Implications of the Studies

The data reported seem to provide encouraging evidence as to the possibility of using microswitch technology with beneficial effects. In particular, the data seem to underline three points, that is, (a) the importance of experimental microswitches to extend the range of responses suitable for microswitch-based programs and thus the number of persons who might benefit from those programs; (b) the importance of using combinations of microswitches to extend the participants' activity, input, and choice opportunities; and (c) the importance of conceiving combinations of microswitches and SGD to promote the participants' activity and interaction.

The studies evaluating new combinations of experimental microswitches and nontypical responses have collected an extensive amount of encouraging evidence as to the possibility of helping most affected persons (i.e., persons who could not possibly be involved in intervention programs relying on typical motor responses and traditional microswitches) (Lancioni et al. 2005c, 2008b). Identifying strategies that offer these persons the possibility to be active and manage their environmental stimulation could represent a breakthrough with multiple implications in terms of educational perspectives and technology development (Lancioni et al. 2010a, 2011; Leung and Chau 2010).

With regard to the educational perspectives, the main point to underline is that persons who were previously excluded from microswitch-based programs or had only marginal access to them may now have a full share of these programs. Their participation in these programs (a) could change their condition from passive recipients of environmental stimulation to active agents practicing self-determination and control with an obvious improvement in social status and quality of life and (b) would substantially modify the conventional educational plans available for them within educational and care contexts (Browder et al. 2001; Karvonen et al. 2004; Lachapelle et al. 2005; Lancioni et al. 2006d, e, 2007d; Petry et al. 2005, 2009; Szymanski 2000; Wehmeyer and Schwartz 1998; Zekovic and Renwick 2003).

With regard to technology development, one would need to underline the importance of upgrading some of the microswitches available and of finding new response-microswitch combinations. Upgrading microswitches may consist of providing more satisfactory designs for the available microswitches or developing new forms of microswitches. One example of the latter is represented by the camera-based technology that allows the possibility of monitoring small responses through the use of one or two color marks rather than through support frames in contact with the participants' face and head (Lancioni et al. 2010a). Finding new response-microswitch combinations may be important to create intervention alternatives that could facilitate the progress of persons only marginally at ease using the combinations available or could create a suitable path for persons unlikely to benefit from any of the combinations available. For example, one could investigate the usability of prolonged eyelid closures for participants for whom this type of response may be much more plausible than double blinks or upward looking (see above) and use adapted optic sensors or camera-based microswitch technology to monitor it. Camera-based technology might also be useful for a response such as minimal tongue movement/ protrusion in a person with virtually no functional movements (Leung and Chau 2010).

The studies targeting multiple responses through multiple microswitches provide a clear view of the wide enrichment potential that microswitch-based programs may have. The use of multiple responses/microswitches, in fact, allows a person to extend the level of activity engagement and to broaden the range of sensory input (preferred stimulation) obtainable. The possibility to obtain different types of stimuli would be expected to increase response motivation and enjoyment. It would also promote choice. In essence, the person would be expected to choose one response over another (or others) if, and as long as, the stimuli related to that response are more highly preferred and the cost of the response is not excessive compared to the cost of the other(s) (Cannella et al. 2005; Stafford et al. 2002). One could easily argue that activity, choice, self-determination, and multiple stimulus input are sufficiently strong variables, capable of promoting a sense of personal fulfillment, improve the person's mood, and ultimately enhance the person's quality of life (Algozzine et al. 2001; Dillon and Carr 2007; Green and Reid 1999; Hoch et al. 2002; Kazdin 2001; Lancioni et al. 2004c, 2006a; Ross and Oliver 2003).

The potential risk of programs involving microswitch-based intervention strategies has been acknowledged. They allow activity and free access to stimulation, but they do not provide opportunities of interaction with the caregiver. The marginality (irrelevance) of this risk in most daily contexts has also been underlined. Together with these clarifications, examples were provided of strategies that could include the opportunity of combining free access to stimulation input and a call function for requesting caregiver's attention. Those strategies rely on the use of microswitches (directly connected to environmental stimulation) and SGD (allowing the person to activate the call function).

Conclusions

The studies reviewed in this chapter underline the importance that microswitches can have within programs for persons with severe/profound intellectual and multiple disabilities. Programs adopting microswitches can help these persons acquire constructive occupation and control access to stimulation independently. Persons with minimal response repertoire can also be successfully introduced in those programs (i.e., through the use of new, experimental microswitches suitable for nontypical responses). The general benefits of the programs may grow considerably if combinations of microswitches (rather than single microswitches) are used. Programs adopting microswitches and SGD technology can help the persons with their occupation, access to stimulation, as well as in ensuring their social contact with the caregiver.

New research initiatives to improve the aforementioned forms of technology and their applications could focus on several issues. For example, one might (a) search for additional nontypical responses and matching microswitches and (b) investigate new solutions to upgrade the microswitch technology already available for monitoring a variety of nontypical responses. One form of technology that might be further upgraded with obvious practical benefits is the camera-based microswitch. This technology could ensure high reliability in monitoring a variety of small (nontypical) responses and would eliminate the need for using more intrusive devices/microswitches on the person's body (e.g., eyeglasses with optic sensors; see Lancioni et al. 2010a; Leung and Chau 2010). One additional issue for research could concern an assessment of when to use multiple microswitches and when to combine microswitches and SGD technology (Lancioni et al. 2008c; Sigafoos et al. 2009).

References

Algozzine, B., Browder, D., Karvonen, M., Test, D. W., & Wood, W. M. (2001). Effects of interventions to promote self-determination for individuals with disabilities. *Review of Educational Research, 71*, 219–277.

Browder, D. M., Wood, W. M., Test, D. W., Karvonen, M., & Algozzine, B. (2001). Reviewing resources on self-determination: A map for teachers. *Remedial and Special Education, 22*, 233–244.

Cannella, H. I., O'Reilly, M. F., & Lancioni, G. E. (2005). Choice and preference assessment research with people with severe to profound developmental disabilities: A review of the literature. *Research in Developmental Disabilities, 26*, 1–15.

Catania, A. C. (2007). *Learning* (4th Interim ed.). New York: Sloan Publishing.

Crawford, M. R., & Schuster, J. W. (1993). Using microswitches to teach toy use. *Journal of Developmental and Physical Disabilities, 5*, 349–368.

Dewson, M. R. J., & Whiteley, J. H. (1987). Sensory reinforcement of head turning with nonambulatory, profoundly mentally retarded persons. *Research in Developmental Disabilities, 8*, 413–426.

Dillon, C. M., & Carr, J. E. (2007). Assessing indices of happiness and unhappiness in individuals with developmental disabilities: A review. *Behavioral Interventions, 22*, 229–244.

Glickman, L., Deitz, J., Anson, D., & Stewart, K. (1996). The effect of switch control site on computer skills of infants and toddlers. *American Journal of Occupational Therapy, 50*, 545–553.

Green, C. W., & Reid, D. H. (1999). A behavioral approach to identifying sources of happiness and unhappiness among individuals with profound multiple disabilities. *Behavior Modification, 23*, 280–293.

Gutowski, S. J. (1996). Response acquisition for music or beverages in adults with profound multiple handicaps. *Journal of Developmental and Physical Disabilities, 8*, 221–231.

Hoch, H., McComas, J. J., Johnson, L., Faranda, N., & Guenther, S. L. (2002). The effects of magnitude and quality of reinforcement on choice responding during play activities. *Journal of Applied Behavior Analysis, 35*, 171–181.

Holburn, S., Nguyen, D., & Vietze, P. M. (2004). Computer-assisted learning for adults with profound multiple disabilities. *Behavioral Interventions, 19*, 25–37.

Karvonen, M., Test, D. W., Wood, W. M., Browder, D., & Algozzine, B. (2004). Putting self-determination into practice. *Exceptional Children, 71*, 23–41.

Kazdin, A. E. (2001). *Behavior modification in applied settings* (6th ed.). New York: Wadsworth.

Lachapelle, Y., Wehmeyer, M. L., Haelewyck, M. C., Courbois, Y., Keith, K. D., Schalock, R., Verdugo, M. A., & Walsh, P. N. (2005). The relationship between quality of life and self-determination: An international study. *Journal of Intellectual Disability Research, 49*, 740–744.

Lancioni, G. E., Bellini, D., Oliva, D., Singh, N. N., O'Reilly, M. F., Lang, R., & Didden, R. (2011). Camera-based microswitch technology to monitor mouth, eyebrow, and eyelid responses of children with profound multiple disabilities. *Journal of Behavioral Education, 20*, 4–14.

Lancioni, G. E., Bellini, D., Oliva, D., Singh, N. N., O'Reilly, M. F., & Sigafoos, J. (2010a). Camera-based microswitch technology for eyelid and mouth responses of persons with profound multiple disabilities: Two case studies. *Research in Developmental Disabilities, 31*, 1509–1514.

Lancioni, G. E., O'Reilly, M. F., & Basili, G. (2001a). An overview of technological resources used in rehabilitation research with people with severe/profound and multiple disabilities. *Disability and Rehabilitation, 23*, 501–508.

Lancioni, G. E., O'Reilly, M. F., & Basili, G. (2001b). Use of microswitches and speech output systems with people with severe/profound intellectual or multiple disabilities: A literature review. *Research in Developmental Disabilities, 22*, 21–40.

Lancioni, G. E., O'Reilly, M. F., Cuvo, A. J., Singh, N. N., Sigafoos, J., & Didden, R. (2007a). PECS and VOCA to enable students with developmental disabilities to make requests: An overview of the literature. *Research in Developmental Disabilities, 28*, 468–488.

Lancioni, G. E., O'Reilly, M. F., Oliva, D., & Coppa, M. M. (2001c). A microswitch for vocalization responses to foster environmental control in children with multiple disabilities. *Journal of Intellectual Disability Research, 45*, 271–275.

Lancioni, G. E., O'Reilly, M. F., Oliva, D., & Coppa, M. M. (2001d). Using multiple microswitches to promote different responses in children with multiple disabilities. *Research in Developmental Disabilities, 22*, 309–318.

Lancioni, G. E., O'Reilly, M. F., Oliva, D., Singh, N. N., & Coppa, M. M. (2002a). Multiple microswitches for multiple responses with children with profound disabilities. *Cognitive Behaviour Therapy, 31*, 81–87.

Lancioni, G. E., O'Reilly, M. F., Sigafoos, J., Singh, N. N., Oliva, D., & Basili, G. (2004a). Enabling a person with multiple disabilities and minimal motor behaviour to control environmental stimulation with chin movements. *Disability and Rehabilitation, 26*, 1291–1294.

Lancioni, G. E., O'Reilly, M. F., Singh, N. N., Buonocunto, F., Sacco, V., Colonna, F., Navarro, J., Lanzilotti, C., Olivetti Belardinelli, M., Bosco, A., Megna, G., & De Tommaso, M. (2009a). Evaluation of technology-assisted learning setups for undertaking assessment and providing intervention to persons with a diagnosis of vegetative state. *Developmental Neurorehabilitation, 12*, 411–420.

Lancioni, G. E., O'Reilly, M. F., Singh, N. N., Buonocunto, F., Sacco, V., Colonna, F., Navarro, J., Oliva, D., Megna, G., & Bosco, A. (2009b). Technology-based intervention options for post-coma persons with minimally conscious state and pervasive motor disabilities. *Developmental Neurorehabilitation, 12*, 24–31.

Lancioni, G. E., O'Reilly, M. F., Singh, N. N., Buonocunto, F., Sacco, V., Colonna, F., Navarro, J., Lanzilotti, C., & Megna, G. (2010b). Post-coma persons with minimal consciousness and motor disabilities learn to use assistive communication technology to seek environmental stimulation. *Journal of Developmental and Physical Disabilities, 22*, 119–129.

Lancioni, G. E., O'Reilly, M. F., Singh, N. N., Campodonico, F., Marziani, M., & Oliva, D. (2004b). A microswitch program to foster simple foot and leg movements in adult wheelchair users with multiple disabilities. *Cognitive Behavior Therapy, 33*, 137–142.

Lancioni, G. E., O'Reilly, M. F., Singh, N. N., Groeneweg, J., Bosco, A., Tota, A., Smaldone, A., Stasolla, F., Manfredi, F., Baccani, S., & Pidala, S. (2006a). A social validation assessment of microswitch-based programs for persons with multiple disabilities employing teacher trainees and parents as raters. *Journal of Developmental and Physical Disabilities, 18*, 383–391.

Lancioni, G. E., O'Reilly, M. F., Singh, N. N., Oliva, D., Baccani, S., Severini, L., & Groeneweg, J. (2006b). Micro-switch programmes for students with multiple disabilities and minimal motor behaviour: Assessing response acquisition and choice. *Pediatric Rehabilitation, 9*, 137–143.

Lancioni, G. E., O'Reilly, M. F., Singh, N. N., Oliva, D., Coppa, M. M., & Montironi, G. (2005a). A new microswitch to enable a boy with minimal motor behavior to control environmental stimulation with eye blinks. *Behavioral Interventions, 20*, 147–153.

Lancioni, G. E., O'Reilly, M. F., Singh, N. N., Oliva, D., & Groeneweg, J. (2003). Using microswitches with persons who have profound multiple disabilities: Evaluation of three cases. *Perceptual and Motor Skills, 97*, 909–916.

Lancioni, G. E., O'Reilly, M. F., Singh, N. N., Oliva, D., Piazzolla, G., Pirani, P., & Groeneweg, J. (2002b). Evaluating the use of multiple microswitches and responses for children with multiple disabilities. *Journal of Intellectual Disability Research, 46*, 346–351.

Lancioni, G. E., O'Reilly, M. F., Singh, N. N., Sigafoos, J., Didden, R., Oliva, D., & Montironi, G. (2007b). Persons with multiple disabilities and minimal motor behavior using small forehead movements and new microswitch technology to control environmental stimuli. *Perceptual and Motor Skills, 104*, 870–878.

Lancioni, G. E., O'Reilly, M. F., Singh, N. N., Sigafoos, J., Didden, R., Oliva, D., Montironi, G., & La Martire, M. L. (2007c). Small hand-closure movements used as a response through microswitch technology by persons with multiple disabilities and minimal motor behavior. *Perceptual and Motor Skills, 104*, 1027–1034.

Lancioni, G. E., O'Reilly, M. F., Singh, N. N., Sigafoos, J., & Oliva, D. (2008a). Microswitch for vocalization responses: Comparing single- versus dual-microphone arrangements for a man with multiple disabilities. *Psychological Reports, 102*, 935–938.

Lancioni, G. E., O'Reilly, M. F., Singh, N. N., Sigafoos, J., Oliva, D., Antonucci, M., Tota, A., & Basili, G. (2008b). Microswitch-based programs for persons with multiple disabilities: An overview of some recent developments. *Perceptual and Motor Skills, 106*, 355–370.

Lancioni, G. E., O'Reilly, M. F., Singh, N. N., Sigafoos, J., Oliva, D., Baccani, S., Bosco, A., & Stasolla, F. (2004c). Technological aids to promote basic developmental achievements by children with multiple disabilities: Evaluation of two cases. *Cognitive Processing, 5*, 232–238.

Lancioni, G. E., O'Reilly, M. F., Singh, N. N., Sigafoos, J., Oliva, D., & Severini, L. (2008c). Enabling two persons with multiple disabilities to access environmental stimuli and ask for social contact through microswitches and a VOCA. *Research in Developmental Disabilities, 29*, 21–28.

Lancioni, G. E., O'Reilly, M. F., Singh, N. N., Sigafoos, J., Tota, A., Antonucci, M., & Oliva, D. (2006c). Children with multiple disabilities and minimal motor behavior using chin movements to operate microswitches to obtain environmental stimulation. *Research in Developmental Disabilities, 27*, 290–298.

Lancioni, G. E., Saponaro, F., Singh, N. N., O'Reilly, M. F., Sigafoos, J., & Oliva, D. (2010c). A microswitch to enable a woman with acquired brain injury and profound multiple disabilities to access environmental stimulation with lip movements. *Perceptual and Motor Skills, 110*, 488–492.

Lancioni, G. E., Singh, N. N., O'Reilly, M. F., Campodonico, F., Oliva, D., & Vigo, C. M. (2005b). Promoting walker-assisted step responses by an adolescent with multiple disabilities through automatically delivered stimulation. *Journal of Visual Impairment and Blindness, 99*, 109–113.

Lancioni, G. E., Singh, N. N., O'Reilly, M. F., La Martire, M. L., Stasolla, F., Smaldone, A., & Oliva, D. (2006d). Microswitch-based programs as therapeutic recreation interventions for students with profound multiple disabilities. *American Journal of Recreation Therapy, 5*, 15–20.

Lancioni, G. E., Singh, N. N., O'Reilly, M. F., & Oliva, D. (2002c). Using a hand-tap response with a vibration microswitch with students with multiple disabilities. *Behavioural and Cognitive Psychotherapy, 30*, 237–241.

Lancioni, G. E., Singh, N. N., O'Reilly, M. F., & Oliva, D. (2005c). Microswitch programs for persons with multiple disabilities: An overview of the responses adopted for microswitch activation. *Cognitive Processing, 6*, 177–188.

Lancioni, G. E., Singh, N. N., O'Reilly, M. F., Oliva, D., Baccani, S., & Canevaro, A. (2002d). Using simple hand-movement responses with optic microswitches with two persons with multiple disabilities. *Research and Practice for Persons with Severe Disabilities, 27*, 276–279.

Lancioni, G. E., Singh, N. N., O'Reilly, M. F., Oliva, D., & Groeneweg, J. (2005d). Enabling a girl with multiple disabilities to control her favorite stimuli through vocalization and a dual-microphone microswitch. *Journal of Visual Impairment and Blindness, 99*, 179–182.

Lancioni, G. E., Singh, N. N., O'Reilly, M. F., Oliva, D., Smaldone, A., Tota, A., Martielli, G., Stasolla, F., Pontiggia, G., & Groeneweg, J. (2006e). Assessing the effects of stimulation versus microswitch-based programmes on indices of happiness of students with multiple disabilities. *Journal of Intellectual Disability Research, 50*, 739–747.

Lancioni, G. E., Singh, N. N., O'Reilly, M. F., & Sigafoos, J. (2009c). An overview of behavioral strategies for reducing hand-related stereotypies of persons with severe to profound intellectual and multiple disabilities. *Research in Developmental Disabilities, 30*, 20–43.

Lancioni, G. E., Singh, N. N., O'Reilly, M. F., Sigafoos, J., Buonocunto, F., Sacco, V., Colonna, F., Navarro, J., Lanzilotti, C., Bosco, A., Megna, G., & De Tommaso, M. (2009d). A technology-assisted learning setup as assessment supplement for three persons with a diagnosis of post-coma vegetative state and pervasive motor impairment. *Research in Developmental Disabilities, 30*, 1034–1043.

Lancioni, G. E., Singh, N. N., O'Reilly, M. F., Sigafoos, J., Buonocunto, F., Sacco, V., Colonna, F., Navarro, J., Megna, G., Chiapparino, C., & De Pace, C. (2009e). Two persons with severe post-coma motor impairment and minimally conscious state use assistive technology to access stimulus events and social contact. *Disability and Rehabilitation: Assistive Technology, 4*, 367–372.

Lancioni, G. E., Singh, N. N., O'Reilly, M. F., Sigafoos, J., Buonocunto, F., Sacco, V., Navarro, J., Addante, L. M., & D'Agostino, I. (2010d). Persons with acquired brain injury and multiple disabilities access stimulation independently through microswitch-based technology. *Perceptual and Motor Skills, 111*, 485–495.

Lancioni, G. E., Singh, N. N., O'Reilly, M. F., Sigafoos, J., Didden, R., Oliva, D., Severini, L., Smaldone, A., Tota, A., & Lamartire, M. L. (2007d). Effects of microswitch-based programs on indices of happiness of students with multiple disabilities: A new research evaluation. *American Journal on Mental Retardation, 112*, 167–176.

Lancioni, G. E., Singh, N. N., O'Reilly, M. F., Sigafoos, J., Oliva, D., Costantini, A., Gatto, S., Marinelli, V., & Putzolu, A. (2006f). An optic microswitch for an eyelid response to foster environmental control in children with minimal motor behaviour. *Pediatric Rehabilitation, 9*, 53–56.

Leatherby, J. K., Gast, D. L., Wolery, M., & Collins, B. C. (1992). Assessment of reinforcer preference in multi-handicapped students. *Journal of Developmental and Physical Disabilities, 4*, 15–36.

Leung, B., & Chau, T. (2010). A multiple camera tongue switch for a child with severe spastic quadriplegic cerebral palsy. *Disability and Rehabilitation: Assistive Technology, 5*, 58–68.

McDougall, J., Evans, J., & Baldwin, P. (2010). The importance of self-determination to perceived quality of life for youth and young adults with chronic conditions and disabilities. *Remedial and Special Education, 31*, 252–260.

Mechling, L. C. (2006). Comparison of the effects of three approaches on the frequency of stimulus activation, via a single switch, by students with profound intellectual disabilities. *The Journal of Special Education, 40*, 94–102.

Petry, K., Maes, B., & Vlaskamp, C. (2005). Domains of quality of life of people with profound multiple disabilities: The perspective of parents and direct support staff. *Journal of Applied Research in Intellectual Disabilities, 18*, 35–46.

Petry, K., Maes, B., & Vlaskamp, C. (2009). Measuring the quality of life of people with profound multiple disabilities using the QOL-PMD: First results. *Research in Developmental Disabilities, 30*, 1394–1405.

Realon, R. E., Favell, J. E., & Dayvault, K. A. (1988). Evaluating the use of adapted leisure materials on the engagement of persons who are profoundly, multiply handicapped. *Education and Training in Mental Retardation, 23*, 228–237.

Ross, E., & Oliver, C. (2003). The assessment of mood in adults who have severe or profound mental retardation. *Clinical Psychology Review, 23*, 225–245.

Sandler, A. G., & McLain, S. C. (1987). Sensory reinforcement: Effects of response-contingent vestibular stimulation on multiply handicapped children. *American Journal of Mental Deficiency, 91*, 373–378.

Saunders, M. D., Smagner, J. P., & Saunders, R. R. (2003). Improving methodological and technological analyses of adaptive switch use of individuals with profound multiple impairments. *Behavioral Interventions, 18*, 227–243.

Schalock, R., Brown, I., Brown, R., Cummins, R. A., Felce, D., Matikka, L., Keith, K. D., & Parmenter, T. (2003). Conceptualization, measurement, and application of quality of life for persons with intellectual disabilities: Reports of an international panel of experts. *Mental Retardation, 40*, 457–470.

Schlosser, R. W., & Sigafoos, J. (2006). Augmentative and alternative communication interventions for persons with developmental disabilities: Narrative review of comparative single-subject experimental studies. *Research in Developmental Disabilities, 27*, 1–29.

Shih, C.-H., Chang, M.-L., & Shih, C.-T. (2010). A new limb movement detector enabling people with multiple disabilities to control environmental stimulation through limb swing with a gyration air mouse. *Research in Developmental Disabilities, 31*, 875–880.

Sigafoos, J., Green, V. A., Payne, D., Son, S. H., O'Reilly, M. F., & Lancioni, G. E. (2009). A comparison of picture exchange and speech-generating devices: Acquisition, preference, and effects on social interaction. *Augmentative and Alternative Communication, 25*, 99–109.

Stafford, A. M., Alberto, P. M., Fredrick, L. D., Heflin, L. J., & Heller, K. W. (2002). Preference variability and the instruction of choice making with students with severe intellectual disabilities. *Education and Training in Mental Retardation and Developmental Disabilities, 37*, 70–88.

Sullivan, M. W., Laverick, D. H., & Lewis, M. (1995). Fostering environmental control in a young child with Rett syndrome: A case study. *Journal of Autism and Developmental Disorders, 25*, 215–221.

Szymanski, L. S. (2000). Happiness as a treatment goal. *American Journal on Mental Retardation, 105*, 352–362.

Wacker, D. P., Wiggins, B., Fowler, M., & Berg, W. K. (1988). Training students with profound or multiple handicaps to make requests via microswitches. *Journal of Applied Behavior Analysis, 21*, 331–343.

Wehmeyer, M. L., & Schwartz, M. (1998). The relationship between self-determination, quality of life, and life satisfaction for adults with mental retardation. *Education and Training in Mental Retardation and Developmental Disabilities, 33*, 3–12.

Zekovic, B., & Renwick, R. (2003). Quality of life for children and adolescents with developmental disabilities: Review of conceptual and methodological issues relevant to public policy. *Disability and Society, 18*, 19–34.

Chapter 3
Speech-Generating Devices for Communication and Social Development

Abstract This chapter provides an overview of studies on using speech-generating devices (SGDs) to improve the communication and social functioning of persons with severe/profound and multiple disabilities. The studies are divided into four groups based on the pragmatic function of the communication responses targeted for improvement. The first group concerns studies that targeted the requesting function. The second group concerns studies on teaching communicative rejecting. The third group consists of studies on developing more socially oriented forms of communication, such as recruiting social interaction and/or initiating conversation. The fourth group includes studies aimed at reducing problem behaviors by teaching functional use of SGDs. The final part of this chapter analyzes the outcomes of the studies reviewed, considers the implications of these findings for overall communication and social development, and highlights directions for future research.

Introduction

Speech-generating devices (SGDs) are a type of assistive technology that can be programmed to produce digitized (i.e., recorded) or synthesized speech output. SGDs are also referred to as voice-output communication aids (VOCAs). A range of SGDs exists: from simple microswitches producing a brief prerecorded message to highly sophisticated computer technologies capable of generating an infinite number of complex utterances via speech synthesis technology (Mullennix and Stern 2010). Commercially available SGDs that exemplify this range of options are shown in Figs. 3.1, 3.2, and 3.3.

SGDs are prescribed as assistive technology aids for individuals who present with severe communication impairment. The term "severe communication impairment" is used to refer to situations where the individual either has (a) highly unintelligible speech, (b) temporarily or permanently lost the ability to speak, or (c) failed

G.E. Lancioni et al., *Assistive Technology: Interventions for Individuals with Severe/Profound and Multiple Disabilities*, Autism and Child Psychopathology Series, DOI 10.1007/978-1-4614-4229-5_3,

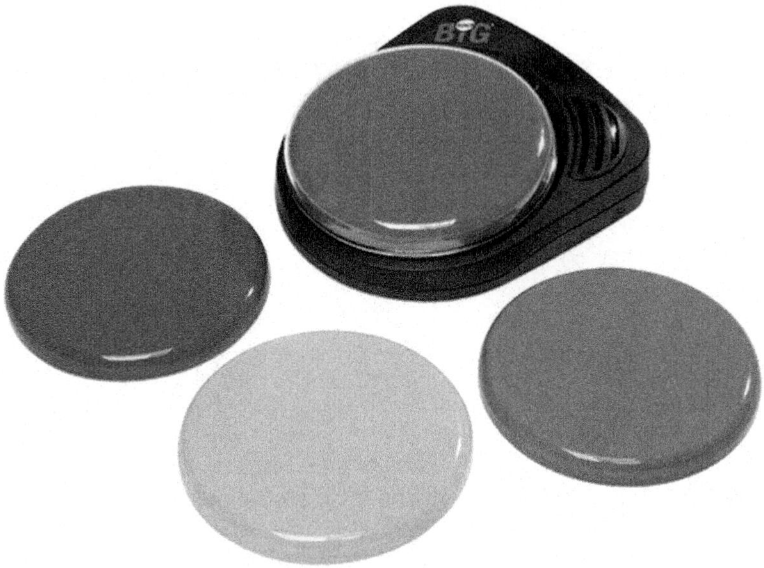

Fig. 3.1 BIGmack switches in various colors. The BIGmack switch is a single-message plate switch that produces digitized (recorded) speech output. The BIGmack is produced by Able Net, Inc. © 1985–2011 AbleNet Inc. All Rights Reserved/Image used with permission

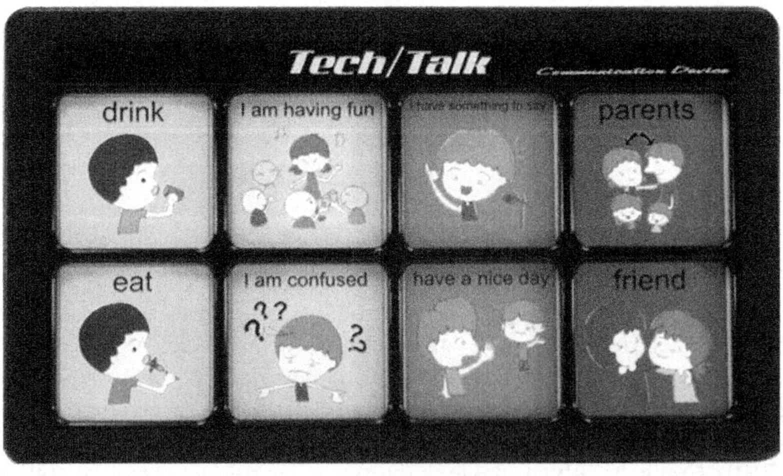

Fig. 3.2 TechTalk SGD. The TechTalk holds overlays of eight symbols/panels and has eight different levels giving it a capacity for up to 64 digitized (recorded) messages. Image used with permission

to develop sufficient speech and language ability to meet his or her everyday communication needs (Hemsley et al. 2001). For such cases, the SGD is intended to augment the person's unintelligible speech or provide an alternative to speech when it has been lost or has failed to develop satisfactorily.

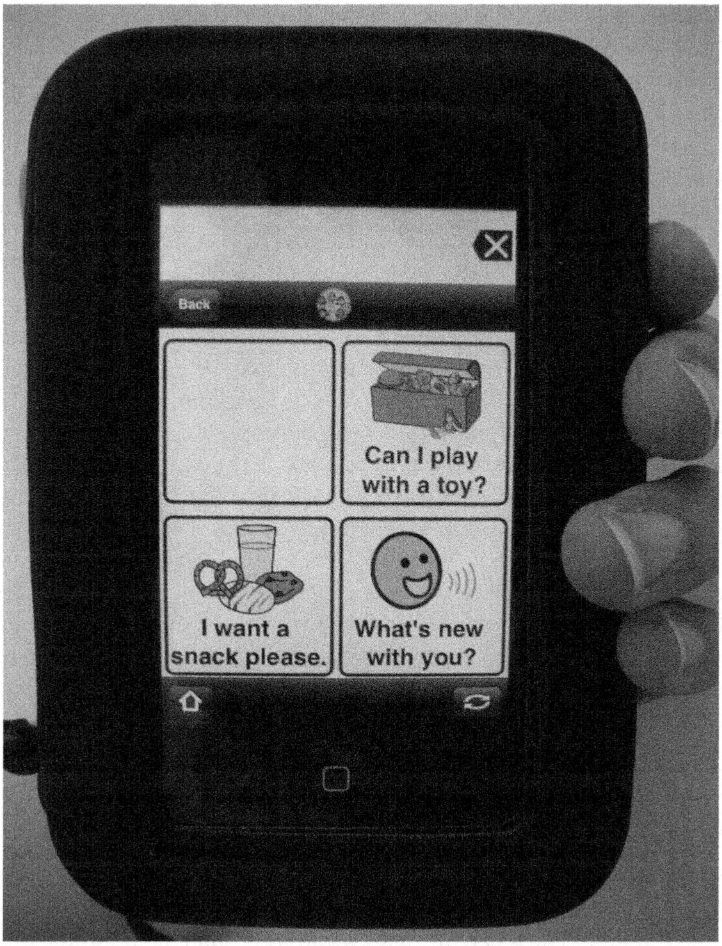
Back
Can I play
with a toy?
I want a
snack please.
What's new
with you?

Fig. 3.3 Photograph of an iPod Touch® that has been configured for use as an SGD. The iPod is placed inside an iMainGo® 2 speaker case to improve sound amplification. The visual display shows three graphic symbols for snacks, toys, and social interaction. Lightly tapping each symbol produces corresponding synthesized speech output (e.g., *can I play with a toy*) that is preprogrammed using Proloquo2Go™ software

Individuals with severe/profound and multiple disabilities can be viewed as potential candidates for SGDs because many such individuals present with severe communication impairment (Matas et al. 1985). These individuals also often have cognitive impairments, which means they are likely to require systematic instruction to learn how to use SGDs for communicative purposes. The potential ramifications of severe communication impairment are far reaching and include (a) limiting the person's ability to express basic wants and needs, (b) restricting opportunities for social interaction, and (c) seriously reducing overall quality of life. There is thus considerable need for effective evidence-based interventions for teaching SGD use. If functional use of SGDs can be taught to persons with severe/profound and multiple disabilities, then SGDs would represent a form of assistive technology that could potentially ameliorate the negative impact of severe communication impairment for such individuals.

SGDs have a number of potential advantages when compared to other AAC options, such as manual signing or picture-exchange communication (Schepis et al. 1996; Schlosser and Blischak 2001). First, the digitized or synthesized speech output from an SGD may provide a more natural and readily interpreted communicative signal. Second, the speech-output feature of SGDs means there is a built-in attention-gaining component when the person activates the device. This, in turn, may increase the probability of listeners attending to the person's communicative attempts. The inherent attention-gaining function may be especially critical to successful communication for individuals with severe/profound and multiple disabilities given that such individuals often lack appropriate attention-gaining skills (Sobsey and Reichle 1989). Third, SGDs can also be programmed to produce very precise messages (e.g., *I need help putting on my shoes*), which may reduce misunderstandings and prevent communicative breakdowns. Fourth, there is evidence that some individuals with developmental disabilities and severe communication impairment may prefer to use SGDs over other AAC options (van der Meer et al. 2011a). In such cases, use of the person's preferred option may increase motivation to learn and use AAC. Fifth, compared to manual signs and picture-exchange systems of AAC, SGDs are considered by some to be perceived as more acceptable and less stigmatizing for the individual and his or her family and friends (Mirenda 2009).

Despite these potential advantages, AAC interventions involving SGDs are likely to be more expensive to set up and more complicated to implement. Thus, it would seem important to critically appraise the available evidence regarding the use of SGDs for improving communicative and social functioning of individuals with severe/profound and multiple disabilities. The aim of this chapter is to review studies that have sought to teach persons with severe/profound and multiple disabilities to use SGDs. This review of intervention studies will consider the type of communication skill targeted for intervention, the type of SGD that was employed, the intervention procedures, and the success of the intervention program.

Successful use of SGDs within habilitation programs for persons with severe/profound and multiple disabilities would seem to require at least two basic conditions to be met. First, the person must have a reliable and efficient way of activating the device. This means that the person must be capable of making a response that will result in selecting the correct icon from the SGD display so as to activate the corresponding speech output. As with the use of microswitches (see Chap. 2), a response form for selecting icons from the display and activating the corresponding speech output should be identified that is either already available in the person's repertoire or which can be taught to the person. In either case, the response should be relatively easy for the person to perform. For persons with sufficient fine motor skills, access will typically involve direct selection, that is, directly pointing to, pressing, or touching switches or panels on the SGD. As shown in Figs. 3.2 and 3.3, the visual displays of SGDs are typically configured with pictures, line drawings, or other types of graphic symbols. The pictures, drawings, or symbols can be seen as having the equivalent status of spoken words or phrases (e.g., touching the picture of an *apple* might produce synthetic speech output such as *I would like to have an apple, please*). For persons who lack sufficient motor skills, access will require some type of switch interface and scanning option, rather than direct selection. For example, some SGDs have a light cursor that will systematically scan the available vocabulary options on the SGD. The person selects a vocabulary option by operating a microswitch (see Chap. 2) when the light lands on the desired option. Scanning with microswitch interfaces is generally slower and more laborious than direct selection (White et al. 2010).

Second, because communication involves a reciprocal interaction between at least two persons (i.e., the SGD user and his or her communicative partner), it is necessary to ensure that the communicative partner responds to the user's SGD-based communication in ways that will reinforce the person's communicative acts and thus motivate him or her to (a) learn use of the SGD to communicate and (b) maintain his or her use of the SGD over time. Related to this latter requirement is the need to ensure the person is taught to use the SGD to produce relevant vocabulary (messages) that will lead to meaningful (i.e., necessary, reinforcing, and relevant) communicative interactions with his or her communicative partners.

To assist rehabilitation professionals in the appraisal of the evidence related to the use of SGDs for individuals with severe/profound and multiple disabilities, this chapter provides an overview of intervention studies that have evaluated the use of SGDs to improve communication and social functioning in this population. To provide a logical organization of this body of evidence, the studies have been divided into four groups based on the communicative function of the target responses. The first group concerns studies that targeted the requesting function. The second group concerns studies on teaching communicative rejecting. The third group consists of studies on developing more socially oriented forms of communication, such as recruiting attention/social interaction and/or initiating conversation. The fourth group includes a brief review of studies aimed at reducing problem behaviors by teaching SGD-based communication as this topic is covered more fully in Chap. 7. The final part of this chapter analyzes the outcomes of the studies reviewed, considers the implications of these findings for overall communication and social development, and highlights directions for future research.

Studies Targeting Communicative Requesting

AAC intervention for individuals with severe/profound and multiple disabilities often begins by teaching individuals to request access to preferred objects or activities. Individuals have also been taught to request help with difficult tasks (McGregor et al. 1992) and to request attention from caregivers (Sobsey and Reichle 1989). As this latter skill is viewed as more socially oriented, studies related to attention-gaining will be covered in the next section on teaching social communication.

With respect to requesting preferred objects/activities, the findings of two recent literature reviews indicate that this communicative function was the most common intervention target in studies focused on teaching SGD use to individuals with autism (van der Meer and Rispoli 2010) and other developmental disabilities (Rispoli et al. 2010). Reichle et al. (1991) delineated several reasons why requesting may be an appropriate initial communicative target for individuals with severe/profound and multiple disabilities. First, requesting is one of the earliest communicative functions to emerge in typically developing children and is thus likely to be a developmentally appropriate goal even for individuals with very low levels of adaptive behavior functioning. Second, requesting access to preferred stimuli is highly functional as it enables the individual to gain reinforcement. This reinforcement might then increase learning and willingness to participate in later intervention sessions that are intended to teach other more socially oriented communication. Third, development of a large repertoire of requesting skills would enable individuals to express their preferences and exert some degree of control over the stimuli that they access, thus going some way toward improving their quality of life. An important question then is whether individuals with severe/profound and multiple disabilities can be successfully taught to use SGDs to make requests for preferred objects and activities.

Table 3.1 lists 23 studies that focused on addressing the question of whether individuals with severe/profound and multiple disabilities can be taught to use SGDs to make requests for preferred objects/activities (Banda et al. 2010; Brady 2000; Dattilo and Camarata 1991; Dyches 1998; Dyches et al. 2002; Gee et al. 1991; Kagohara et al. 2010; Kozleski 1991; Lancioni et al. 2001; Locke and Mirenda 1988; Mechling and Cronin 2006; Romski et al. 1988; Russell and Beard 1992; Schepis and Reid 1995; Schepis et al. 1996, 1998; Sigafoos and Drasgow 2001; Sigafoos et al. 2004a; Sigafoos et al. 2004c; Soto et al. 1993; Van Acker and Grant 1995; van der Meer et al. 2011b; Wacker et al. 1988). These studies are summarized in Table 3.1 in terms of the number of participants, participant age, the type of SGD used, and the types of symbols used in conjunction with the SGD, if this information was provided. To illustrate the range of SGDs used and the intervention approaches taken within this set of 23 studies, we next provide a detailed description of six representative studies from Table 3.1.

First, Locke and Mirenda (1988) provided intervention to an 11-year-old boy with severe/profound intellectual disability. The child was also blind and had no speech. The aim of the intervention was to teach the child to request six preferred foods and drinks by pressing one of six texture symbols. These symbols were attached to a keyboard overlay connected to an Apple IIe computer with Talking Word Board software that provided speech output. Pressing one of the textured symbols generated a prestored message (e.g., *potato chip*). An A-B design (Kennedy 2005) was implemented in the school setting and used to evaluate the effects of intervention. During the first A (baseline) phase, all six preferred items were named by the trainer and the child was allowed to touch and smell them. However, the child was not prompted to press the symbols, and no reinforcement was given if he did so. At the beginning of the B (intervention) phase, the child was physically assisted to

Table 3.1 Studies on teaching individuals to use SGD to request preferred objects/activities

Studies	Participants	Age	SGD device/symbol system
Locke and Mirenda (1988)	1	11	Computer/texture symbols
Romski et al. (1988)	4	14–19	Computer keyboard/lexigrams
Wacker et al. (1988)	6	12–20	Tape recorder via a microswitch
Dattilo and Camarata (1991)	2	21–36	TouchTalker/Minspeak software
Gee et al. (1991)	3	5–10	Switch-operated call buzzer
Kozleski (1991)	2	6, 15	Switches/photographs
Russell and Beard (1992)	1	10	PowerPad switch/picture
Soto et al. (1993)	1	22	Wolf/Sigsymbols
Schepis and Reid (1995)	1	23	MegaWolf/photographs
Van Acker and Grant (1995)	3	5–11	Computer/line drawings
Schepis et al. (1996)	3	23–42	MegaWolf, MessageMate/photographs
Dyches (1998)	4	10–12	BigRed, JellyBean, CheapTalk8/ photographs
Schepis et al. (1998)	4	3–5	CheapTalk/black and white symbols
Brady (2000)	2	5, 5	Microswitches/line drawings
Lancioni et al. (2001)	1	9	Microswitches
Sigafoos and Drasgow (2001)	1	14	BIGmack/Picture Communication Symbols
Dyches et al. (2002)	1	17	Speakeasy/Picture Communication Symbols
Sigafoos et al. (2004a)	2	16, 20	BIGmack/Picture Communication Symbols
Sigafoos et al. (2004c)	1	12	TalkTrac/Boardmaker drawings
Mechling and Cronin (2006)	3	17–21	Level Communicator/photographs
Banda et al. (2010)	2	17, 21	TechTalk/photographs
Kagohara et al. (2010)	1	17	iPod Touch/Proloquo2Go software
van der Meer et al. (2011a)	3	13–23	iPod Touch/Proloquo2Go software

touch each texture symbol to orient him to the presence of these symbols and to the speech-output message generated when each texture was pressed. During intervention, every time the child pressed a texture symbol and generated the corresponding speech output, he was given a small amount of the corresponding preferred item. He also received spoken feedback from the trainer (*Oh, you want a potato chip*). If the child did not press a symbol independently, he was physically prompted to do so. Prompting consisted of a slight nudge to move his arm toward the keyboard overlay. Initially, only one or two textures were placed on the overlay. New texture symbols were added after the child had made five independent requests. This process continued until all six texture symbols had been added to the overlay. After intervention, generalization probes were conducted during a group snack activity. Contingent reinforcement and prompting were used during these probes. The results suggested that the intervention procedures were effective in teaching the child to use the texture-symbol SGD. Specifically, during baseline, no independent requests occurred. With intervention, there was a gradual but steady increase in the number of unprompted requests. Unprompted requests also occurred during the generalization probes. There are two unique aspects to this study that warrant comment. First, to compensate for the child's visual impairment, the researchers developed a unique set of texture-based symbols (e.g., wool, velvet) with each texture representing a different food or drink item (e.g., juice, cereal). Second, verbal prompting was never used, and thus, it would appear that the child learned to make requests that were controlled by the mere presence of the preferred items. One potential limitation of this study is that the child did not appear to require symbol discrimination training. Other children, however, might not associate different textures with specific items and may thus require additional symbol discrimination training, which could prolong and complicate the intervention process. Another limitation is the A-B design, which is preexperimental and thus fails to adequately control for extraneous variables, such as history, exposure, practice, and maturation (Kennedy 2005), although it is unlikely that these variables would have been responsible for the child's rapid acquisition of the targeted requesting responses. Despite these limitations, this is an important study because it appears to be the first to have taught SGD use to a child who not only had severe/profound intellectual disability but who was also blind.

Second, Gee et al. (1991) worked with three boys who were 5, 7, and 10 years of age, respectively. The boys were described as having severe/multiple disabilities. The aim of the study was to teach the boys to make a generalized request (i.e., want) using a switch-operated call buzzer. With this device, a tone, buzzer, or tape-recorded message was produced when the switch was pressed. Thus, similar to Locke and Mirenda (1988), the boys were taught to use a direct selection response. The study was conducted in the context of four classroom routines (i.e., recess, lunch, using a blender, and toy play). The objective of the intervention was to teach the boys to make a request, by touching the switch, when the ongoing routine was interrupted. A multiple-probe across subjects design (Kennedy 2005) was used to evaluate the effects of the intervention. During baseline, the trainer interrupted the activity and waited 5 or 10 s for the child to make a request. A request could involve activating the SGD or use of gestures or vocalizations. During intervention, progressive time delay and decreasing levels of physical assistance were used to prompt SGD use (Duker et al. 2004). Specifically, when the activity was interrupted, the children were initially given immediate and full physical assistance to activate the SGD. Activations were reinforced by enabling the activity to continue, which was presumed to be a reinforcer. Over successive interruptions, physical assistance was delayed and its magnitude reduced. The consequence of continuing the activity did in fact appear to function as reinforcement for these boys in that independent requests using the SGD increased during the intervention phase. Interestingly, as the boys learned to use the SGD, their use of gesture requests tended to decrease, suggesting that these responses were replaced by the newly acquired responses of activating the SGD. Because the children's informal gestures were likely to be less readily interpreted by unfamiliar listeners, this finding is important in showing that existing, but less effective communicative requests, can be replaced by teaching children to use SGDs.

Third, Schepis et al. (1996) provided intervention to two women and one man who were 23, 42, and 38 years of age, respectively. These three adults were described as having profound intellectual disability, and they were also nonambulatory due to physical impairment (i.e., spastic quadriplegia). The participants lived in a residential center, and the intervention program took place in a training room at the participants' habilitation unit within the center with additional postintervention sessions conducted in the participants' living rooms, a snack shop, and the home of a friend. The aim of the intervention was to teach the participants to request access to preferred objects and activities by selecting photographs affixed to SGDs. Prior to the intervention, a preference assessment was undertaken to identify four preferred items for each participant (e.g., cookies, magazines, and milk). Color photographs were made of each preferred item and affixed to a MegaWolf or MessageMate SGD. When a photograph was selected, the SGD produced corresponding output (*I want the [item/activity], please*) in either digitized (MessageMate) or synthesized speech (MegaWolf). Again, the SGDs were operated via direct selection, that is, by pressing on a photograph affixed to the device. The study involved a sequence of baseline, training, and posttraining phases with training and posttraining phases introduced in a staggered multiple-baseline fashion across participants and across items/activities within participants. During baseline sessions, each of which consisted of five opportunities to request, the trainer initiated each opportunity by approaching the participant, asking *What do you want?* and waiting 15 s to see if the participant would activate the SGD. During the training phase, the trainer used a 15-s time delay and graduated guidance (Duker et al. 2004) to prompt SGD-based requests from the participants. Requests were then reinforced by providing the requested item or activity. The procedures in place during the posttraining phase were identical to baseline except trained and untrained items were included for the participants to request. Compared to baseline, all three participants showed an increase in the use of their SGD to make requests as a function of the training procedures. The increase was largely maintained during posttraining and during probes in other settings and with other untrained items/activities, although two of the three participants never requested new, untrained items during the posttraining phase. The results showed that the participants learned to make specific requests using the SGDs with the implementation of systematic instructional procedures (i.e., graduated guidance and time delay). An important finding in this study was that use of the SGD generalized to settings where no training had occurred. This is an important finding from a habilitation perspective because it suggests that training in the use of SGDs may enable individuals to communicate across a range of settings and not just in those settings where explicit instruction is provided.

Fourth, Sigafoos et al. (2004a) described an intervention aimed at teaching two students with developmental disabilities to use SGDs when their initial and gesture-based communicative attempt was unsuccessful. That is, SGDs were used as a way of repairing a communicative breakdown. The study provided intervention to one male and one female participant who were 16 and 20 years old, respectively. The participants had severe intellectual disability and autism/pervasive developmental disorder. The female (older participant) also had bilateral hearing loss. Neither participant had any speech, although they could make vocalizations (e.g., screaming, whining, humming). They could also indicate when they wanted something by simple gestures, such as reaching for or leading a person's hand to a desired object. The study was conducted in a self-contained classroom at a private school for students with disabilities. The study involved baseline and intervention phases that were staggered in accordance with a multiple-baseline across subjects design (Kennedy 2005). Prior to baseline, a number of preferred foods were identified for the participants using a systematic preference assessment (Duker et al. 2004). The SGD used in the study was a BIGmack switch (AbleNet, Inc.). The switch was affixed with a black and white line drawing representing *WANT* from the Mayer-Johnson Picture Communication Symbols Combination Book (Mayer-Johnson Co. 1994). Operating this device involved putting approximately three ounces of pressure on the top of the switch, which then activated a prerecorded message (i.e., *I want more*). During each baseline and intervention session, participants received six opportunities to request preferred foods. During baseline, the participant could gain access to a tray of preferred foods by using gestures (reaching, leading) or by using the SGD. For five of the six opportunities, whichever response occurred first was reinforced by giving the participant access to the tray of preferred foods. For the sixth trial, however, use of gestures was ignored for 10 s to determine if the participant would attempt to repair this communicative breakdown by using the SGD. Because SGD use was not observed in baseline, intervention procedures were implemented to teach the participants to use the SGD when a communicative breakdown occurred (i.e., when the use of gestures was ignored). The results showed that use of the SGD to repair communicative breakdowns increased as a function of the intervention and eventually occurred during 80–100 % of the communicative breakdowns for both participants. This finding suggests that SGD use might represent a viable repair strategy. More generally, teaching effective repair strategies is an important habilitation goal because communicative breakdowns are frequently experienced by individuals with severe disabilities (Brady and Halle 2002).

Fifth, Banda et al. (2010) described a novel, video-based procedure for teaching two participants to operate SGDs to request preferred objects. The participants were two men aged 17 and 21 years. Both had autism and no functional speech, although the older participant produced "prosodic jargon." The study occurred in the participant's special education classrooms and involved baseline, video modeling, and generalization phases that were arranged in a multiple-baseline across subjects design (Kennedy 2005). Prior to baseline, preferred (e.g., chips, pudding) and nonpreferred (clipboard, paper napkins) items were identified using a systematic preference assessment (Duker et al. 2004). Photographs of the preferred and nonpreferred items were affixed to the panels of a Tech/Talk SGD. During baseline the SGD was available, but participants were not prompted to use it. Next, video modeling was implemented, which consisted of showing participants a 10–15-s video clip showing an adult activating the SGD to request preferred objects. Participants then had the opportunity to use the SGD. The video clip was repeated if participants failed to use the SGD within 15 s. Sessions continued for up to 30 min or until the acquisition criterion was met (i.e., 80 % SGD use). Following the video-modeling intervention, generalization probes were conducted for a second untrained item, but otherwise following the baseline procedures. The results showed that correct SGD use increased for both participants during the video-modeling intervention, although gains were relatively modest and below the acquisition criteria for one participant and neither participant used the SGD during the 1- and 3-week generalization probes. While the use of video modeling is an innovative approach for teaching individuals to use SGDs to request preferred items, the results of the present study suggest that this teaching approach may need to be combined with more direct response prompting to promote acquisition and generalization.

Sixth, van der Meer et al. (2011b) sought to determine whether three individuals with developmental disabilities could learn to use an iPod-based SGD to request preferred foods and leisure materials. Three individuals with severe intellectual disability (aged 13, 14, and 23 years) participated. All three had severely impaired speech development, which was limited to a few single words. The study was conducted in the participants' special educational classroom at a school that catered to adolescents and young adults with developmental disabilities. The SGD consisted of an Apple iPod Touch with Proloquo2Go software that produced synthesized speech output. Each participant's iPod was configured with three colored line drawings representing snacks, toys, and social interaction (see Fig. 3.3). Touching each graphic produced corresponding speech output (i.e., *I want a snack, please, Can I play with a toy?* and *What's new with you?*). Baseline, acquisition training, posttraining, and follow-up sessions were arranged in a multiple-baseline across subjects design (Kennedy 2005). The aim of acquisition training was to teach participants to request preferred snacks or toys by touching the correct icon. One participant preferred both snacks and toys and was thus taught to request both, but the other two only preferred snacks and so they received training only on snacks. During baseline sessions of 5-min duration, preferred items were offered and each instance of correct SGD use was recorded. For acquisition training, a discrete-trial training approach was used (Duker et al. 2004). For each trial, an item was offered. If a correct request did not occur within 10 s, graduated guidance (Duker et al. 2004) was used to prompt a request and then the person received access to the preferred items. The posttraining phase and then the 10-week follow-up sessions occurred once participants reached the acquisition criterion (i.e., three successive unprompted requests). These final phases were identical to baseline, except that access to preferred items occurred only when the participant used the SGD. Two of the three participants reached the acquisition criteria within ten trials, indicating rapid acquisition. These two individuals continued to make requests with the SGD, and without prompting, at rates that averaged from two to five responses per minute during both the posttraining and follow-up sessions. The third participant failed to achieve acquisition and thus did not progress to posttraining. The results suggest that the instructional approach was effective in teaching successful use of the iPod-based SGD for two of the three participants, but that modified procedures may be required to ensure others achieve acquisition. Still, the data suggest that some individuals with severe disabilities can be successfully taught to use iPods as SGDs.

When considered collectively, the outcomes of these 23 studies were largely positive in that most participants learned to use the SGDs to make the targeted requests. However, a minority of participants showed little or no progress when intervention to teach SGD-based requesting was implemented. Still, the results for most of the participants in the studies summarized in Table 3.1 provide evidence that there are effective instructional procedures available for teaching individuals with severe/profound and multiple disabilities to use SGDs to make requests for preferred objects and activities. These largely positive findings suggest that SGDs are viable options for some such individuals at least for use in a beginning AAC intervention where the focus is on teaching requests for preferred objects/activities. However, the database has so far been limited to relatively simple responses (i.e., direct selection of a line drawing by pressing a panel on the SGD) and requests for preferred food, drinks, or toys/activities. There appear to be no studies on teaching individuals with severe/profound and multiple disabilities to use SGDs to request assistance, for example. Along those lines, McGregor et al. (1992) taught a 20-year-old man to use a TouchTalker with Minspeak software to request help with vocational tasks, but this participant had moderate disabilities and his SGD was intended to augment his existing, albeit largely unintelligible, speech. Future research should focus on teaching SGD use to individuals who are unable to make direct selections and thus require some sort of scanning approach to activate the SGD. Teaching requests for more abstract and distant reinforcers (e.g., requesting community-based activities) and requesting sequences that require more complicated multiple response/symbol activations are additional areas for future research.

Studies Targeting Communicative Rejecting

Another early intervention target when beginning an AAC program for individuals with severe/profound and multiple disabilities is the acquisition of responses that enable the individual to communicate a desire to escape from or avoid nonpreferred objects and activities. For example, the person might need to be taught to produce a voice-output message of *No thanks* when offered a nonpreferred beverage. As with requesting, there are several reasons why rejecting is an appropriate initial communicative target for individuals with severe/profound and multiple disabilities. First, rejecting emerges early in typically developing children and is thus developmentally appropriate for individuals at the beginning stages of AAC intervention (Sigafoos et al. 2002). Second, rejecting nonpreferred objects and activities is functional in enabling the individual to gain [negative] reinforcement and avoid aversive (nonpreferred) stimulation (Sigafoos et al. 2004b). Third, development of socially appropriate rejecting skills enables individuals to communicate that they do not want something. This ability can be seen as one way to foster greater self-determination and improve overall quality of life. An important question then is whether individuals with severe/profound and multiple disabilities can be successfully taught to use SGDs to reject nonpreferred or unwanted objects and activities.

Table 3.2 lists three studies that have focused on addressing the question of whether individuals with severe/profound and multiple disabilities can be taught to use SGDs to reject nonpreferred objects/activities (Choi et al. 2010; Lancioni et al.

Table 3.2 Studies on teaching individuals to use SGD to reject nonpreferred objects/activities

Studies	Participants	Age	SGD device/symbol system
Sigafoos and Roberts-Pennell (1999)	1	6	Switch with digitized speech
Lancioni et al. (2006)	2	9, 12	Microswitches with yes/no output
Choi et al. (2010)	3	6–9	TechSpeak, Springboard, Vantage with yes/no icons/output

2006; Sigafoos and Roberts-Pennell 1999). These studies are summarized in Table 3.2 in terms of the number of participants, participant age, the type of SGD used, and the types of symbols used in conjunction with the SGD.

Sigafoos and Roberts-Pennell (1999) provided intervention to two 6-year-old boys with severe intellectual disability. Their speech and language abilities were estimated at the 10-month level. One of these children was taught to use an SGD due to the fact that he resisted being prompted to shake his head. The other child was taught to indicate a reject by shaking his head *no* as he showed no such resistance to prompting, and this gesture was considered a natural way to indicate a reject. The study was conducted in the children's special education classroom and included baseline, intervention, generalization, and follow-up phases arranged in a multiple-baseline across subjects design (Kennedy 2005). Each baseline session consisted of six discrete trials. For each trial, the child was offered a pair of items consisting of a more preferred (e.g., chips) and a less preferred (e. g., water) item. The items were offered, and the child allowed to choose one item by reaching for it. When the child reached for an item, the trainer then either gave the child that item or attempted to give the child the other [wrong] item (i.e., the item that the child had not reached for/chosen). The aim of the subsequent intervention phase was to teach the children to reject the wrong item when it was offered. Intervention involved the trainer giving the child the wrong item and then waiting 3, 5, or 10 s for the child to produce a correct rejecting response. If a correct rejecting response did not occur, a series of prompts (verbal, gesture, physical) was implemented. A correct rejecting response for one child involved shaking his head *no*. For the other child, a correct rejecting response involved pressing the switch, which then produced the message *No thanks. I want the other one.* When a correct rejecting response occurred, the wrong item was removed and the child received the correct item. Generalization probes involved presenting the children with two new pairs of more and less preferred items that had not been used during the intervention phase. A new trainer also conducted some of these sessions to access generalization across people. Follow-up sessions, using the same procedures as the generalization phase, occurred at 2 weeks and 3 or 4 months later. The child who was taught to use the SGD consistently performed in the 80–100 % correct range after eight intervention sessions. This high level of performance generalized to new pairs of items and to a new trainer and was maintained at the 2-week and at the 3- and 4-month follow-up sessions. Results for the child who was taught to use the headshake gesture were similar. Thus, both children learned to reject the wrong item. The authors concluded that this "wrong-item" format can be used as a context for teaching AAC-based rejecting responses to children with severe disabilities who lack speech. However, the study is confounded somewhat by the fact that after rejecting the wrong item, children received the [more preferred] item. Thus, the task would appear to have included elements of both rejecting and requesting. Still, this study is important in that it demonstrated successful intervention procedures for teaching a 6-year-old child to use an SGD to reject wrong (i.e., nonchosen or mismatched) items.

Lancioni et al. (2006) provided SGD training to one boy and one girl, who were 9 and 12 years of age, respectively. The children had severe/profound intellectual disability, physical disability (spastic tetraparesis), and visual impairment. Preferred (e.g., chips, music, tea) and nonpreferred (sparkling water, sponge, scarf) stimuli were identified. The program aimed to teach the children to indicate *yes* when offered a preferred item and to indicate *no* when offered a nonpreferred item. The novel aspect of this study was the manner in which the children were enabled to indicate *yes* and *no*. This involved providing each child with a microswitch arrangement linked to an SGD. The arrangement allowed for two response options producing vocal output of either *yes* or *no*. Baseline, intervention, and postintervention sessions were arranged in a multiple-baseline across subjects design (Kennedy 2005). During baseline, the children were offered a stimulus and asked *Do you want this?* The item offered was removed following 15 s or if the child activated the SGD via the microswitch arrangement. For intervention, children were again offered stimuli as in baseline, but a correct *yes* (or *no*) response led to presentation (or removal) of the stimulus. A response was prompted using physical guidance if it did not occur within 15 s of stimulus presentation. The same procedures were in place during the postintervention phase except additional preferred and nonpreferred stimuli were presented. The results showed that activation of the microswitches to produce *yes* and *no* output increased from very low levels in baseline to very high levels during the intervention and postintervention phase. In addition, both children eventually achieved a high level (above 75 % correct) of response discrimination in that they correctly produced *yes* when presented with a preferred stimulus and *no* when presented with a nonpreferred stimulus. These results suggest that the microswitch-based SGD set-ups were acquired relatively quickly by the two children. The study demonstrated the acquisition of an important yes/no discrimination. Such a discrimination is required in many everyday communicative interactions. The finding that this important discrimination generalized to a large number of new stimuli increases the applied relevance of the study.

The final study in this group involved four boys (6–9 years of age) with developmental disabilities/autism and severe communication impairment (Choi et al. 2010). Three of the four children were taught to use SGDs. The fourth child was taught to use a nonelectronic picture-exchange communication system. The three SGD users were provided with different devices (i.e., Vantage, Tech Speak, or Springboard). These devices were configured with icons for requesting a missing item and for indicating a communicative reject when offered a wrong item. For example, pressing a *DVD* icon was used to request a missing DVD, whereas pressing the *NO* icon was used to indicate that they had received the wrong item. The study was conducted in the children's self-contained special education classrooms and involved pretraining, baseline, training, generalization, and follow-up phases. These phases were arranged in a multiple-baseline across subjects design (Kennedy 2005). Pretraining was used to ensure the children could access the materials needed to engage in a preferred activity. For example, to drink some juice, the child required a straw or to watch a movie, the child required a DVD. When the required item was missing, children were expected to request that item and this then provided the trainer with the opportunity to deliver either the correct missing item (matched trails) or deliver a different [wrong] item (mismatched trials). The principle aim of the study was to teach the children to reject the offer of the wrong item on mismatched trials. In baseline, children received the two types of trials (matched vs. unmatched) in which the child received either the requested or nonrequested (wrong) item. Once presented, the trainer waited 10 s to see if the children would use their AAC system (i.e., SGD or picture-exchange) to reject the wrong item. The training phase was intended to teach this skill by prompting the children to emit the correct rejecting response when offered the wrong item. Prompting involved the trainer tapping the correct icon and then fading this prompt by waiting increasing amounts of time before prompting (i.e., progressive time delay, Duker et al. 2004). Generalization probes occurred in the context of new activities, and follow-up sessions occurred 2 weeks after the last generalization probe. The three children using SGDs showed rapid progress in learning to request the missing item and then make a rejecting response if they received the wrong item. The fourth child, who used the picture-exchange system, required intensive training before he mastered this requesting/rejecting sequence. The newly acquired responses also generalized and maintained at generally high levels (above 75 %) for the three SGD users, but occurred at lower percentages for the fourth child. The results replicate and extend the findings of Sigafoos and Roberts-Pennell (1999) on the use of the wrong-item format for teaching children with developmental disabilities to use SGDs to reject nonchosen or nonrequested items. Interestingly, the results showed better acquisition with the SGDs than the picture-exchange system, although it is important to note that the study was not specifically designed to compare SGDs with picture-exchange communication.

As an intervention target for individuals with severe/profound and multiple disabilities, communicative rejecting has been subject to much less research than communicative requesting (Sigafoos et al. 2004b). Still, the outcomes of the three studies summarized in Table 3.2 are largely positive in that all of the participants provided with SGDs learned to use their respective devices to make the targeted rejecting responses. Overall, then the studies summarized in Table 3.2 provide some evidence that individuals with severe/profound and multiple disabilities can be taught to use SGDs to reject less preferred or wrong items. However, the existing database is limited in terms of (a) the number and ages of participants, (b) the number and types of rejecting responses that have been taught, and (c) the context in which those rejecting responses have been taught. Contexts studied so far have been discrete opportunities where a nonpreferred or wrong item has been offered. Future research should focus on teaching persons to use SGDs to make more varied types of rejecting responses as well as teaching related communication skills, such as protesting and indicating negation.

Studies Targeting Social Communication

The third group of studies includes interventions aimed at teaching individuals with severe/profound and multiple disabilities to use SGDs for more socially oriented communication exchanges. Socially oriented communication includes (a) recruiting the attention of a listener and (b) initiating conversation. Acquisition of social communication is a priority for individuals with severe/profound and multiple disabilities for two main reasons. First, the ability to recruit attention and initiate conversational exchanges is often severely hindered due to severely impaired speech and language development (Reichle et al. 1991; Sobsey and Reichle 1989). Thus, teaching these skills addresses a common deficit area. While individuals with severe/profound and multiple disabilities may have some existing informal and prelinguistic acts to recruit attention (e.g., moving toward a person, vocalizing), such behaviors often fail to be recognized as an attempt to communicate, and thus, these acts might either decrease in frequency (i.e., extinction) or escalate to problematic forms, such as tantrums, aggression, or self-injury (Sigafoos et al. 2006). In addition, informal and prelinguistic behaviors are often too nonspecific to function as effective ways of initiating conversational exchanges. Thus, individuals with severe/profound and multiple disabilities might benefit from learning to use SGDs to recruit attention and initiate conversation because such devices can be programmed to produce specific and naturalistic speech output. Such messages are, in turn, perhaps more likely to be recognized and responded to that existing informal prelinguistic acts. Second, while teaching requesting and rejecting is important in enabling individuals to exert control over access to objects and activities, recruiting attention and initiating conversations brings the person into the world of others. Without such skills, the person may remain socially isolated and consequently suffer a reduced quality of life. An important question then is whether individuals with severe/profound and multiple disabilities can be successfully taught to use SGDs to recruit attention and initiate conversational exchanges. Unlike requesting and rejecting, socially oriented communication would seem more abstract and less directly linked to tangible reinforcement. Thus, there may be cognitive and motivational aspects that could make the teaching of social communication more difficult. A review of the evidence on this issue follows.

Table 3.3 lists 22 studies that focused on addressing the question of whether individuals with severe/profound and multiple disabilities can be taught to use SGDs to recruit attention and initiate conversations (Adamson et al. 1992; Beck et al. 2009; Bellon-Harn and Harn 2008; Blischak and Lloyd 1996; Buzolich et al. 1991; Cosby and Johnston 2006; Healy 1994; Koppenhaver et al. 2001; Lancioni et al. 2008a, 2008b, 2009a, 2009b, 2009c; Mathy-Laikko et al. 1989; O'Keefe and Dattilo 1992; Schweigert 1989; Sobsey and Reichle 1989; Spiegel et al. 1993; Thunberg et al. 2009a, 2009b; Trembath et al. 2009; Trottier et al. 2011). These studies are summarized in Table 3.3 in terms of the number of participants, participant age, the type of SGD used, and the types of symbols used in conjunction with the SGD. We next describe six of these studies in detail to illustrate the range of SGDs and proce-

Table 3.3 Studies on teaching individuals to use SGD to recruit social interaction/initiate conversation

Studies	Participants	Age	SGD device/symbol system
Mathy-Laikko et al. (1989)	1	8	Four switches/texture symbols
Schweigert (1989)	1	7	Microswitch linked to call buzzer
Sobsey and Reichle (1989)	6	6–16	Switch with buzzer output
Buzolich et al. (1991)	3	9–12	LightTalker, TouchTalker, AudTalker
Adamson et al. (1992)	12	6–20	Computer w/Words+/Lexigrams
O'Keefe and Dattilo (1992)	3	24–60	TouchTalker with Minspeak software
Spiegel et al. (1993)	1	19	TouchTalker with Minspeak software
Healy (1994)	1	17	ScanWolf/line drawings
Blischak and Lloyd (1996)	1	35	AllTalk/graphic symbol overlays
Koppenhaver et al. (2001)	6	3–7	BIGmack, CheapTalk/line drawings
Cosby and Johnston (2006)	3	3–4	Single-switch SGD
Bellon-Harn and Harn (2008)	1	6	Hawk/pictures
Lancioni et al. (2008a)	3	10–15	Microswitches linked to SGD
Lancioni et al. (2008b)	2	16, 18	Microswitches linked to SGD
Beck et al. (2008)	2	25, 35	Go-Talk 20/pictures
Lancioni et al. (2009a)	2	32, 33	Microswitches linked to SGD
Lancioni et al. (2009b)	11	5–18	Microswitches linked to SGD
Lancioni et al. (2009c)	8	5–17	Microswitches linked to SGD
Thunberg et al. (2009a)	4	5–7	TechTalk 2, Clicker 3
Thunberg et al. (2009b)	3	5–7	Clicker 3
Trembath et al. (2009)	3	3–5	Talara-32/Boardmaker symbols
Trottier et al. (2011)	2	11, 11	Vantage, Springboard/Boardmaker symbols

dures that have been developed and evaluated for enhancing the social communication skills of individuals with severe/profound and multiple disabilities.

First, Mathy-Laikko et al. (1989) conducted an assessment/intervention study involving an 8-year-old girl with profound intellectual disability, cortical blindness, and moderate hearing loss. The study had multiple objectives, but the main aim was to teach the child to use an SGD to recruit attention from care staff in her residential facility. The SGD consisted of four switches, each of which could be covered in a different texture (i.e., velvet, cloth, sandpaper, aluminum). The child received sessions of approximately 60 min each 5 days per week. The study involved three sequential phases: (a) baseline, (b) surface preference, and (c) social contingency. During baseline, the child was presented with the four switches, but each switch had the same smooth surface (i.e., the textures had not yet been applied to the switch faces). When a switch was pressed, it produced the message *Hello [child's name]* via a Votrax speech synthesizer. The child was never prompted to press any of the switches in baseline. During the surface preference phase, each switch was covered with a different texture. As in baseline, pressing a switch produced the message *Hello [child's name]*. The purpose of this phase was to determine if the child showed a preference for touching one or more of the textures. In the final [social contingency] phase, pressing the preferred textured switch resulted in a new message

[Staff person's name], please come and play with me. Upon hearing this message, the staff person approached the child, placed the child's hand on the switch again, and then interacted socially with the child for 15–25 s. During this final phase, pressing any of the other three switches produced the previous message (*Hello [child's name]*). At a later point, a different texture/switch was paired with the new message and social contingency. Data were collected on the frequency with which each switch was pressed in each phase. The results showed that the frequency of switch pressing in baseline ranged from means of 6.3 to 14.8. During the surface preference phase, the frequency of switch pressing increased and the child most often activated the switch with the velvet texture, suggesting a preference for touching this texture. In the final social contingency phase, use of the switch associated with recruiting attention was more frequent compared to the other phases and other switches. However, it is important to note that there was a considerable amount of variability in the frequency of responding. Still, the results suggest that the child did learn to operate a simple, switch-based SGD to recruit attention/social contact from staff.

Second, Buzolich et al. (1991) sought to increase social communication in three children (aged 9–12 years) with cerebral palsy and intellectual disability. Three SGD were used, one for each participant: (a) LightTalker, (b) TouchTalker, and (c) AudTalker. Ten social vocabulary/messages were programmed into each device (e.g., *It was fun, Sounds good, I liked it*). The children received daily 45-min sessions in their classroom with other children and teachers attending. The effects of intervention were evaluated in a multiple-baseline across subjects design (Kennedy 2005). The children received pretraining to ensure they could activate their respective SGD. During baseline, opportunities for social communication were provided by asking questions. The percentage of opportunities with an appropriate SGD-based comment by participants was recorded, but participants were never prompted to use the SGD. During intervention, if participants did not use the SGD to converse when an opportunity arose, a least-to-most prompting procedure (Duker et al. 2004) was implemented, which consisted of looking expectantly, waiting 10 s, indirect verbal prompt (e.g., *What could you say?*), direct verbal prompt (e.g., *You could say it was fun*), and modeling use of the SGD. The results suggest the intervention was eventually effective in that three participants reached the 80 % correct level in 2, 15, and 19 intervention sessions, respectively. These gains were largely maintained for two of the three participants. The findings suggest that some individuals might require a considerable amount of direct prompting to spontaneously engage in these types of social-communicative acts with an SGD.

Third, Healy (1994) described the results of an intervention that was implemented with a 17-year-old male with severe intellectual disability, cerebral palsy, and no speech. The adolescent was provided with a ScanWolf that produced synthesized speech output. Line drawing symbols representing single words and short phrases were configured as vocabulary choices on the SGD. The aim of the intervention was to teach the participant to initiate conversations and respond to the initiations of teachers, school staff, and peers. Data were collected during baseline and intervention sessions of 15-min duration that occurred during three activities (i.e., group activities, recess, and lunch) in his special education setting. A multiple baseline across these three activities (Kennedy 2005) was used to evaluate the effects of the intervention. Prior to baseline, the participant received four 30-min pretraining sessions during which he was taught to operate the SGD. During baseline, the participant had his previous communication board that contained line drawings, single words, and short phrases. During intervention, he was provided with the SGD fitted with an overlay containing 36 line drawings, single words, and short phrases as in baseline. The results showed less than three initiations per session in baseline. Initiations increased during intervention by one to three responses with the introduction of the SGD. These results suggest that the pretraining and provision of the SGD lead to increased conversation initiation, although the increase seemed to be context specific in that initiations were higher during recess and group activities than during lunch. This latter finding could stem from competing behavior (i.e., eating) during lunch. While lunch may be the ideal time to teach requesting and rejecting, this finding suggests that professionals should consider the context in which to target increases in SGD-based social communication.

Fourth, Cosby and Johnston (2006) provided a single-switch SGD to three children with severe, multiple disabilities in an attempt to increase their social-communicative interactions with their typically developing peers. The children ranged from 3 years 6 months to 6 years 6 months of age. The study was undertaken in the children's kindergarten classrooms that included children with and without disabilities. The SGD was programmed with two phrases (*That looks like fun. Can I play?*) and placed in locations that were easily accessible to the children. Baseline, intervention, and maintenance phases were arranged in a multiple-baseline across subjects design (Kennedy 2005). For each phase, observers recorded the number of times each child used the SGD when an opportunity to initiate using the preprogrammed message arose during each 20–45-min session. During baseline, the children were in the classroom with toys available and the teacher engaged the child in some interaction. The SGD was present, but children were never instructed to use it. For intervention, typical peers in the classroom were told that the target children might use the SGD to initiate a social interaction and the peers should respond positively to any such use by incorporating the target child into their social interaction. The target children were also prompted to use the SGD when a peer approached. Prompting consisted of physical assistance. For the maintenance phase, the procedures were similar to intervention, except prompting of SGD use did not occur. The results showed that SGD use was low in baseline (one response per session), increased to four to five responses in intervention, and were generally maintained at this level following intervention, although only two of the three children received maintenance sessions. Interestingly, data showed that the typical peers generally responded positively to SGD use by the target children. These findings are important in showing naturalistic use of SGDs by young severely handicapped children and correspondingly appropriate responses to SGD messages by their typically developing peers. However, it is possible that the target children used the SGD to access toys rather than interaction with peers as both consequences often occurred following SGD use.

Fifth, Lancioni et al. (2008a) worked with three students who were 10, 11, and 15 years old. These students had severe to profound intellectual disability, physical disability necessitating wheelchair use (i.e., spastic tetraparesis), and no speech. Each participant was provided with a microswitch system that was linked to an SGD. Different response topographies for closing the microswitch and activating the SGD were identified for each participant. For example, one participant activated the SGD by putting pressure on a switch that was affixed to the back of the wheelchair seat. Once activated, the SGD was programmed to emit phrases such as *Can someone play with me?* that were intended to enable participants to recruit attention/social interaction. The study followed a multiple-baseline design across three target behaviors (Kennedy 2005). Only one of the target behaviors was related to SGD use. The remaining two activated other microswitches that enabled the person to directly obtain preferred sources of stimulation (music, vibration). In baseline, participants had the equipment (microswitches linked to SGDs), but their responses did not produce speech output. For intervention, speech-output messages were produced by each activation of the SGD via the microswitch and a familiar caregiver responded to every third SGD output by interacting socially with the participant. The results showed very few SGD responses (less than 10 per session) during baseline, but these increased to above 20 on average during intervention and remained at this higher level during two postintervention checks. This study is significant in demonstrating the combined use of three microswitches to directly obtain stimulation and to indirectly recruit staff attention/social interaction. The increase in the latter response suggests the participants were motivated to obtain social-communicative interaction and that the microswitch-linked SGDs were an effective form of assistive technology for enabling this to happen.

Sixth, Beck et al. (2009) described a novel, naturalistic approach for developing social communication in SGD users. Their study included one man and one woman who were 25 and 35 years old. Both had developmental disability and were largely nonverbal, except for some vocalizations and gestures. The aim of the program was to increase participants' use of an SGD to initiate conversation and respond to initiations from others. The SGD was a Go-Talk 20 with pictures corresponding to conversational messages. Intervention occurred in the context of 30-min group music sessions that occurred twice per week for 8 weeks. During sessions, staff followed a script and modeled SGD use in addition to speech. Participants were prompted to use the SGD using a 3-s delayed prompting procedure (Duker et al. 2004). All SGD responses by participants were followed by the staff person making a relevant conversational reply. Both participants increased their SGD-initiated conversations during the course of intervention. While this naturalistic approach has appeal for teaching social communication, the present study did not include sufficiently rigorous experimental controls to determine whether the naturalistic approach was in fact responsible for the gains observed.

The outcomes of these 22 studies were largely positive in that most participants learned to use the SGD to recruit attention, initiate conversations, or engage in related social-communicative acts. However, in many cases, the amount of intervention required to teach SGD-based social communication could be viewed as intensive. This might be expected given the severe/multiple impairments experienced by these participants and the fact that most had no previous experience with SGDs.

The need for intensive intervention might also indicate that it could be more difficult to teach social communication to persons with severe/profound and multiple disabilities, as compared to requesting and rejecting.

Still, the results for most of the participants in the studies summarized in Table 3.3 provide evidence that there are effective instructional procedures available for teaching individuals with severe/profound and multiple disabilities to use SGDs to recruit attention and initiate conversations. These are important skills for enhancing the person's social interactions, and SGD-based methods would seem to represent the most natural alternative when the person lacks sufficient speech and language for these and other types of social interactions. Future research should focus on teaching individuals to use SGDs for more complex and sophisticated social communication, such as maintaining conversations and responding to more complex types of questions/initiations from others.

Studies Targeting Reduction of Problem Behavior

This section reviews six studies involving SGDs and functional communication training (Durand 1990). Functional communication training is a procedure for replacing problem behaviors by focusing on the development of functionally equivalent communication (Sigafoos et al. 2009). For example, if the person engages in self-injury to escape from or avoid nonpreferred activities, the logic of functional communication training would indicate the need to teach the person more acceptable ways to reject nonpreferred activities (Durand 1999). Table 3.4 summarizes six studies that have used SGDs and functional communication training as a treatment of problem behavior among individuals with severe/profound and multiple disabilities. Chapter 7 provides a comprehensive review of studies involving the use of assistive technologies in the treatment of problem behaviors.

For example, Durand (1993) worked with three boys who were from 3.5 to 15 years of age. These children were diagnosed with moderate to severe intellectual disability and cerebral palsy. None of the three had any speech, but they did engage in serious problem behaviors (e.g., hair pulling, self-injury, hitting others) that were hypothesized to serve one of three communicative functions. The study was undertaken in the children's classrooms. Observations of 30 min occurred once per week

Table 3.4 Studies on using SGD-based interventions in the treatment of problem behavior

Studies	Participants	Age	SGD device/symbol system
Durand (1993)	3	3–15	Wolf, Introtalker
Sigafoos et al. (1996)	1	11	Switch-operated tape player
Durand (1999)	5	3–15	Introtalker
Olive et al. (2008)	1	4	Four-button Touch Talk
Sigafoos et al. (2008)	1	12	BIGmack/line drawing for *WANT*
Franco et al. (2009)	1	7	Go-Talk/photographs

in the context of various conditions (e.g., one-to-one instruction, group setting, and when the child was alone). The study involved two phases. In the first phase, the children were assessed using the Motivation Assessment Scale (Durand 1990) to identify the variables thought to control each child's problem behavior. The results confirmed the perception that their problem behaviors served one of the following three communicative functions for the three respective children: (a) reject nonpreferred activities and recruit attention [child 1], (b) reject nonpreferred tasks [child 2], and request access to preferred foods [child 3]. Next, intervention was provided with the aim of replacing problem behavior by teaching the children to use SGD to reject, request, and/or recruit attention, respectively. Intervention involved teaching the children to use a Wolf or Introtalker SGD that was programmed with replacement messages (e.g., *I want more* was intended to replace problem behavior related to requesting food, and *I want to take a break* was intended to replace problem behavior related to rejecting nonpreferred tasks). The intervention procedures involved using verbal and physical prompts to use the SGD under the same conditions that evoked problem behavior. The effects of the intervention were evaluated in a multiple-baseline across subjects design (Kennedy 2005). None of the children used their respective SGDs during baseline. Instead, they engaged in problem behavior during an average of 41 [child 1], 14 [child 2], and 67 % [child 3] of the observation intervals. With intervention, unprompted SGD use increased and problem behavior decreased by at least 78 % for each child. The collateral reduction in problem behavior as SGD use increased suggested that the newly acquired SGD-based communication skills came to replace the children's problem behavior. This study appears to be the first to show that problem behavior of children with intellectual, physical, and severe communication impairment can be treated effectively by teaching them to use SGD.

Sigafoos et al. (1996) described an SGD-based intervention for an 11-year-old boy with severe intellectual disability and physical disability necessitating use of a wheelchair. The child also had a visual field deficit in his right eye. He was referred for treatment due to frequent self-injurious head banging, which had been persistent for 10 years and had caused a permanent welt on his forehead. His head banging occurred at high rates on a daily basis. The study involved an initial assessment followed by SGD training. The assessment involved recording the percentage of 10-s intervals with head banging during 5-min sessions. Sessions occurred over 3 days under each of six classroom conditions: (a) academic task, (b) social interaction, (c) making a drink, (d) toy play, (e) sitting outside, and (f) alone. The results showed that head banging occurred at 0 % or 5 % of the intervals during the first five conditions, but was almost constant (90 % of intervals) during the alone condition. This pattern suggested that the child found being alone aversive and thus engaged in head banging to recruit attention from the teacher. This hypothesis is supported by the fact that he would cease his head banging when the teacher approached and interacted with him. Given this hypothesis, the intervention involved teaching him to use an SGD to recruit attention/social interaction from others. The SGD consisted of a switch linked to a tape recorder. Pressing the switch produced the message *Come here, please*. To teach the child to use the SGD, the trainer left him alone for initially a very short time (e.g., 3 s) while he was physically prompted by another person to press the switch. When the message was produced, the trainer returned and engaged the child in a social interaction (e.g., talking to him, interactive toy play). Physical prompting was faded by having the second person wait longer and longer before prompting and eventually being out of the room and out of the child's sight. The effects of this prompting procedure on the child's independent use of the SGD and head banging were evaluated in an ABAB reversal design (Kennedy 2005). The child learned to use the SGD without prompting within 35 training trails (i.e., within seven 5-min sessions), and the child continued to use the SGD on 80–100 % of the opportunities across the remaining 20 sessions. As independent use of the SGD increased, head banging showed a collateral decrease. The results suggest that use of the SGD replaced head banging as the more probable response for recruiting attention. However, the results of this study are limited due to the fact that the researchers did not assess generalization to additional adults nor to less structured sessions. In addition, the study is limited because follow-up data could not be collected due to the ending of the school year. Still, the results show rapid reduction of severe, persistent self-injury by application of a relatively simple SGD-based intervention.

A third illustrative study from this final group involved a 7-year-old child with autism and no speech (Franco et al. 2009). The problem behavior of concern was inappropriate, disruptive vocalizations. A prior assessment indicated that these vocalizations appeared to function as requests for preferred objects and to reject nonpreferred activities. The child was thus provided with a Go-Talk SGD that was programmed with relevant phrases (*I want a break* and *Come with me*) indicated by photograph symbols (e.g., photograph of a stop sign was paired with the *I want a break* message). The child's problem behaviors were observed under conditions when he was involved in four activities (e.g., playing with toys, working on task, being offered preferred items, and interacting with an adult) and either had or did not have the SGD. Results showed that problem behavior was much lower when he had the SGD to use. In addition to reductions in problem behavior, his engagement increased when he had the SGD to use. These positive changes appear to be attributable to the child's newly developed abilities to request breaks from nonpreferred activities and request preferred items, which were made possible by the SGD. It is important to note, however, that the child did receive training to use the SGD, which involved direct physical prompting, reinforcement, and use of a constant 5-s time-delay procedure to fade prompts (Duker et al. 2004).

Discussion

Outcome of the Studies

Overall, the 54 studies summarized in this chapter reported generally positive results. While some participants failed to show much progress, most of the participants in these studies did acquire the skills to use SGDs and used their SGDs successfully for the targeted communication function, be it requesting, rejecting, initiating conversation, or recruiting attention/social interaction. These generally positive findings suggest that SGDs are viable forms of assistive [communication] technology for persons with severe/profound and multiple disabilities. This conclusion is consistent with the findings of three systematic reviews into the use of SGDs for individuals with autism (van der Meer and Rispoli 2010), developmental disabilities (Rispoli et al. 2010), and adults with intellectual disabilities (Sutherland et al. 2010).

Implications for Practice

This generally positive conclusion has several implications for practice. The first is the apparent need for careful, systematic, and often intensive intervention to teach SGD use. The studies examined in this chapter, as well as those in the previous reviews referenced above, suggest that mere provision of an SGD is not sufficient to ensure successful use of such devices for functional communication. Rather, the individuals in these studies all received systematic instruction before they came to use their respective SGDs for functional communication. And before they received systematic instruction (i.e., during baseline) functional use of SGDs was largely absent. The systematic instructional procedures used in these studies varied, but shared a number of generic components:

1. Creating structured opportunities for communication, such as by offering preferred items to request.
2. Prompting SGD use by applying one or more response-prompting strategies, such as graduated guidance.
3. Fading the use of response prompts to promote independent SGD use, such as by the use of time-delay procedures.
4. Providing reinforcement, that is, ensuring listeners responded to SGD activations in ways that functioned to reinforce the person's SGD use.

These types of instructional strategies have been empirically validated for teaching a range of skills to persons with severe/profound and multiple disabilities (Duker et al. 2004; Snell and Brown 2006). Successful outcomes from the application of such strategies are likely to depend on how well the procedures are implemented. Effective implementation of systematic instructional strategies could be conceptualized as another type of [assistive] technology, that is, a technology of systematic instruction (Green and Sigafoos 2007). The implication is that successful use of SGDs to enhance the communication and social development of persons with severe/profound and multiple disabilities would appear to require two types of [assistive] technology. The first type is the careful selection and provision of an SGD that can be operated easily given the cognitive, sensory, and physical capabilities of the individual. The second type involves the effective application of well-established instructional strategies to teach the person to use the SGD for communication purposes. Rehabilitation professionals will thus require competence in selecting SGDs for individuals and competence in designing and implementing behavioral teaching strategies to ensure individuals learn to use their newly prescribed SGD for a range of communication and social purposes.

A second implication arising from our summary and analysis of these 54 studies is that, by establishing the potential viability of SGDs as communication aides for individuals with severe/profound and multiple disabilities, there may be increased application of such devices in AAC interventions for this population. SGDs are also likely to become more widely prescribed because of their purported advantages over other AAC systems, as delineated in the Introduction to this chapter. When these potential advantages are bolstered by additional empirical demonstrations of successful use, it is likely that SGDs will become more widely recommended as communication aids for individuals with severe/profound and multiple disabilities.

However, because some SGDs are relatively more expensive and complicated to program and use than manual signs or picture-exchange AAC, there would seem to be a critical need to carefully match individuals to specific SGDs. Along these lines, consideration should be given to the characteristics of the individual, his or her communicative partners, and the environments in which communication will occur (Sigafoos and Iacono 1993). For example, individuals with visual impairment may require larger or textured symbols, which will impact on the type of overlay that will be needed on the SGD. Similarly, ambulatory persons may require more portable SGDs compared to individuals who use wheelchairs. Additional factors to consider include the (a) nature, length, and number of messages that can be stored in the SGD; (b) intelligibility and volume of speech output; (c) output options (e.g., speech plus printed output); and (d) skills required to operate the device.

However, even careful consideration of such factors offers no guarantee that the selected SGD will be one that the person is capable of learning and interested in using. Consequently, Sigafoos et al. (2005) recommended that individuals receive exposure to a number of different devices (or AAC systems) and that this exposure includes a period of intervention with each device or system. Following this intervention trial, the individual could then be enabled to choose the device or system they would prefer to continue to learn to use. In line with this recommendation, research reviewed by van der Meer et al. (2011a) indicated that individuals with developmental disabilities often show a preference for using one type of AAC system over another (e.g., picture-exchange vs. SGD). When an SGD is the preferred option, Sigafoos et al. (2005) further showed that the participants showed an idiosyncratic preference for using one type of SGD over another. One implication is that individuals may be able to self-determine their own AAC system. This self-determination could be facilitated by a two-step process that involves (a) first teaching them to use several devices and then (b) creating opportunities for them to choose which one of these several devices they would prefer to use.

A third implication is the corresponding need for parents, teachers, and clinicians to gain competence in programming and maintaining the hardware and software of such devices. From our experience, this requires gaining technical literacy and access to ongoing support from technically literate professionals. Another implication that may arise if more individuals are recommended for SGDs is the need to ensure their communicative partners can in fact function as effective listeners. Most potential listeners are unlikely to have had any exposure to someone who uses an SGD. This implies the need to support communicative partners to ensure they are responsive to people who use SGDs.

Future Research Directions

A number of future research directions can be proposed in light of this analysis and summary of studies. First, one might speculate that speech output from SGDs could influence acquisition of communication skills or the responsiveness of listeners. There has been little research into these issues, and it is thus an obvious area for future research. Second, it is possible that speech output from an SGD could facilitate receptive and/or expressive speech as suggested by Blischak et al. (2003) and Romski and Sevcik (1993, 1996). Schlosser et al. (2009) examined the empirical literature on the possibility that output from SGDs could influence natural speech production. They concluded that in some, but not all, cases, SGD output does seem to have a modestly facilitative effect. However, they cautioned that there were currently too few studies investigating this issue to draw any firm conclusions. Thus, the effect of speech output from SGDs on receptive and expressive speech remains equivocal. In the requesting study of van der Meer et al. (2011b), the researchers anecdotally noted that one participant seemed to show an increase in spoken words during the posttraining sessions when he was using an iPod with synthesized speech output to request toys and snacks. However, the words he spoke (e.g., *basketball, outside*) did not match the speech output emanating from the iPod, and the design of the study did not permit the apparent increase in natural speech production to be attributed to use of the iPod-based SGD. Still, one might speculate that there might be ways of using SGDs during communication intervention that could possibly facilitate receptive and expressive speech development among individuals with developmental disabilities who present with little or no pretreatment speech. Counterintuitively, Sigafoos et al. (2011) demonstrated an increase in natural speech production when previously reinforced SGD-based requests were put on extinction (i.e., when such requests were no longer reinforced). However, this study was limited to one adolescent who already had a spoken vocabulary of several single words. Still, the results are intriguing in suggesting the need for more research to understand how best to use SGDs within more comprehensive intervention programs to develop the communication and social skills of individuals with severe/profound and multiple disabilities.

Conclusion

The studies reviewed in this chapter suggest the viability of using SGDs in AAC interventions for individuals with severe/profound and multiple disabilities. Through the application of systematic instructional procedures, persons with severe/profound and multiple disabilities have been successfully taught to use a range of SGDs to (a) make requests for preferred objects and activities, (b) reject nonpreferred (or wrong) objects and activities, and (c) recruit attention/initiate social interaction. SGDs have also been successfully used as part of treatments aimed at reducing problem behaviors. Successful use of SGDs hinges on the quality of instruction provided. Instruction should be based on systematic instructional strategies that have been empirically validated for teaching persons with severe/profound and multiple disabilities. Effective procedures exist for guiding instruction to teach persons to use SGDs to (a) request preferred objects/activities, (b) reject nonpreferred (and wrong) objects/activities, (c) recruit attention, and (d) initiate social interactions. Rehabilitation professionals require skills in selecting SGDs and teaching functional use of such devices. More research is needed to develop effective procedures for teaching other types of communication skills and for teaching more complicated responses beyond selecting a single symbol from an SGD. Future research is also needed on the effect of speech-output technology on the acquisition of communication skills, responsiveness of listeners, and on receptive and expressive speech and language development.

References

Adamson, L. B., Romski, M. A., Deffebach, K., & Sevcik, R. A. (1992). Symbol vocabulary and the focus of conversations: Augmenting language development for youth with mental retardation. *Journal of Speech and Hearing Research, 35*, 1333–1343.

Banda, D. R., Copple, K. S., Koul, R. K., Sancibrian, S. L., & Bogschutz, R. J. (2010). Video modelling interventions to teach spontaneous requesting using AAC devices to individuals with autism: A preliminary investigation. *Disability and Rehabilitation, 32*, 1364–1372.

Beck, A. R., Stoner, J. B., & Dennis, M. (2009). An investigation of aided language stimulation: Does it increase AAC use with adults with developmental disabilities and complex communication needs? *Augmentative and Alternative Communication, 25*, 42–54.

Bellon-Harn, M. L., & Harn, W. E. (2008). Scaffolding strategies during repeated storybook reading: An extension using a voice output communication aid. *Focus on Autism and Other Developmental Disabilities, 23*, 112–124.

Blischak, D. M., & Lloyd, L. L. (1996). Multi-modal augmentative and alternative communication: Case study. *Augmentative and Alternative Communication, 12*, 37–46.

Blischak, D. M., Lombardino, L. J., & Dyson, A. T. (2003). Use of speech-generating devices: In support of natural speech. *Augmentative and Alternative Communication, 19*, 29–35.

Brady, N. C. (2000). Improved comprehension of object names following voice output communication aid use: Two case studies. *Augmentative and Alternative Communication, 16*, 197–204.

Brady, N. C., & Halle, J. W. (2002). Breakdowns and repairs in conversation between beginning AAC users and their partners. In J. Reichle, D. R. Beukelman, & J. C. Light (Eds.), *Exemplary practices for beginning communicators: Implications for AAC* (pp. 323–351). Baltimore: Paul H. Brookes.

Buzolich, M. J., King, J. S., & Baroody, S. M. (1991). Acquisition of the commenting function among system users. *Augmentative and Alternative Communication, 7*, 88–99.

Choi, H., O'Reilly, M., Sigafoos, J., & Lancioni, G. (2010). Teaching requesting and rejecting sequences to four children with developmental disabilities using augmentative and alternative communication. *Research in Developmental Disabilities, 31*, 560–567.

Cosby, J. E., & Johnston, S. (2006). Using a single-switch voice output communication aid to increase social access for children with severe disabilities in inclusive classrooms. *Research and Practice for Persons with Severe Disabilities, 31*, 144–156.

Dattilo, J., & Camarata, S. (1991). Facilitating conversation through self-initiated augmentative communication treatment. *Journal of Applied Behavior Analysis, 24*, 369–378.

Duker, P., Didden, R., & Sigafoos, J. (2004). *One-to-one training: Instructional procedures for learners with developmental disabilities*. Austin: Pro-Ed.

Durand, V. M. (1990). *Severe behavior problems: A functional communication training approach*. New York: Guilford Press.

Durand, V. M. (1993). Functional communication training using assistive devices: Effects on challenging behavior and affect. *Augmentative and Alternative Communication, 9*, 168–176.

Durand, V. M. (1999). Functional communication training using assistive devices: Recruiting natural communities of reinforcement. *Journal of Applied Behavior Analysis, 32*, 247–267.

Dyches, T. T. (1998). Effects of switch training on the communication of children with autism and severe disabilities. *Focus on Autism and Other Developmental Disabilities, 13*, 151–162.

Dyches, T. T., Davis, A., Lucido, B. R., & Young, J. R. (2002). Generalization of skills using pictographic and voice output communication devices. *Augmentative and Alternative Communication, 18*, 124–131.

Franco, J. H., Lang, R. L., O'Reilly, M. F., Chan, J. M., Sigafoos, J., & Rispoli, M. (2009). Functional analysis and treatment of inappropriate vocalizations using a speech-generating device for a child with autism. *Focus on Autism and Other Developmental Disabilities, 24*, 146–155.

Gee, K., Graham, N., Goetz, L., Oshima, G., & Yoshioka, K. (1991). Teaching students to request the continuation of routine activities by using time delay and decreasing physical assistance in the context of chain interruption. *Journal of the Association for Persons with Severe Handicaps, 16*, 154–167.

Green, V. A., & Sigafoos, J. (2007). Overview. In J. Sigafoos & V. A. Green (Eds.), *Teaching and technology* (pp. 1–6). New York: Nova.

Healy, S. (1994). The use of synthetic speech output communication aid by a youth with severe developmental disability. In K. Linfoot (Ed.), *Communication strategies for people with developmental disabilities: Issues from theory and practice* (pp. 156–176). Baltimore: Paul H. Brookes.

Hemsley, B., Sigafoos, J., Balandin, S., Forbes, R., Taylor, C., Green, V. A., & Parmenter, T. (2001). Nursing the patient with severe communication impairment. *Journal of Advanced Nursing, 35*, 827–835.

Kagohara, D. M., van der Meer, L., Achmadi, D., Green, V. A., O'Reilly, M. F., Mulloy, A., Lancioni, G. E., Lang, R., & Sigafoos, J. (2010). Behavioral intervention promotes successful use of an iPod-based communication device by an adolescent with autism. *Clinical Case Studies, 9*, 328–338.

Kennedy, C. H. (2005). *Single-case designs for educational research*. Boston: Allyn and Bacon.

Koppenhaver, D. A., Erickson, K. A., Harris, B., McLellan, J., Skotko, B. G., & Newton, R. A. (2001). Storybook-based communication intervention for girls with Rett syndrome and their mothers. *Disability and Rehabilitation, 23*, 149–159.

Kozleski, E. B. (1991). Expectant delay procedure for teaching requests. *Augmentative and Alternative Communication, 7*, 11–19.

Lancioni, G. E., O'Reilly, M. F., Oliva, D., & Coppa, M. M. (2001). Using multiple microswitches to promote different responses in children with multiple disabilities. *Research in Developmental Disabilities, 22*, 309–318.

Lancioni, G. E., Singh, N. N., O'Reilly, M. F., Sigafoos, J., Oliva, D., & Baccani, S. (2006). Teaching "yes" and "no" responses to children with multiple disabilities through a program including microswitches linked to a vocal output device. *Perceptual and Motor Skills, 102*, 51–61.

Lancioni, G. E., O'Reilly, M. F., Singh, N. N., Sigafoos, J., Oliva, D., & Severini, L. (2008a). Three persons with multiple disabilities accessing environmental stimuli and asking for social contact through microswitch and VOCA technology. *Journal of Intellectual Disability Research, 52*, 327–336.

Lancioni, G. E., O'Reilly, M. F., Singh, N. N., Sigafoos, J., Oliva, D., & Severini, L. (2008b). Enabling two persons with multiple disabilities to access environmental stimuli and ask for social contact through microswitches and a VOCA. *Research in Developmental Disabilities, 29*, 21–28.

Lancioni, G. E., O'Reilly, M. F., Singh, N. N., Sigafoos, J., Didden, R., Oliva, D., Campodonico, F., de Pace, C., Chiapparino, C., & Groeneweg, J. (2009a). Persons with multiple disabilities accessing stimulation and requesting social contact via microswitch and VOCA devices: New research evaluation and social validation. *Research in Developmental Disabilities, 30*, 1084–1094.

Lancioni, G. E., O'Reilly, M. F., Singh, N. N., Sigafoos, J., Oliva, D., Smaldone, A., La Martire, M. L., Antonucci, M., De Pace, C., & Chiapparino, C. (2009b). Persons with multiple disabilities access stimulation and contact the caregiver via microswitch and VOCA technology. *Life Span and Disability, XII*, 119–128.

Lancioni, G. E., Singh, N. N., O'Reilly, M. F., Sigafoos, J., Buonocunto, F., Sacco, V., Colonna, F., Navarro, J., Oliva, D., Signorino, M., & Megna, G. (2009c). Microswitch- and VOCA-assisted programs for two post-coma persons with minimally conscious state and pervasive motor disabilities. *Research in Developmental Disabilities, 30*, 1459–1467.

Locke, P. A., & Mirenda, P. (1988). A computer-supported communication approach for a child with severe communication, visual, and cognitive impairments: A case study. *Augmentative and Alternative Communication, 4*, 15–22.

Matas, J., Mathy-Laikko, P., Beukelman, D., & Legresley, K. (1985). Identifying the nonspeaking population: A demographic study. *Augmentative and Alternative Communication, 1*, 17–31.

Mathy-Laikko, P., Iacono, T., Ratcliff, A., Villarruel, F., Yoder, D., & Vanderheiden, G. (1989). Teaching a child with multiple disabilities to use a tactile augmentative communication device. *Augmentative and Alternative Communication, 5*, 249–256.

Mayer-Johnson Co. (1994). *Picture communication symbols combination book*. Solano Beach, CA: Mayer-Johnson Co.

McGregor, G., Yopung, J., Gerak, J., Thomas, B., & Vogelsberg, R. (1992). Increasing functional use of an assistive communication device by a student with severe disabilities. *Augmentative and Alternative Communication, 8*, 243–250.

Mechling, L. C., & Cronin, B. (2006). Computer-based video instruction to teach the use of augmentative and alternative communication devices for ordering at fast-food restaurants. *Journal of Special Education, 39*, 234–245.

Mirenda, P. (2009). Promising interventions in AAC for individuals with autism spectrum disorders. *Perspectives on Augmentative and Alternative Communication, 18*, 112–113.

Mullennix, J., & Stern, S. (Eds.). (2010). *Computer synthesized speech technologies: Tools for aiding impairment*. Hershey: Medical Information Science Reference.

O'Keefe, B. M., & Dattilo, J. (1992). Teaching the response-recode form to adults with mental retardation using AAC systems. *Augmentative and Alternative Communication, 8*, 224–233.

Olive, M., Lang, R., & Davis, T. (2008). An analysis of the effects of functional communication training and a voice output communication aid for a child with autism spectrum disorder. *Research in Autism Spectrum Disorders, 2*, 223–236.

Reichle, J., York, J., & Sigafoos, J. (1991). *Implementing augmentative and alternative communication: Strategies for learners with severe disabilities*. Baltimore: Paul H. Brookes Publishing Co.

Rispoli, M. J., Franco, J. H., van der Meer, L., Lang, R., & Hoher Camargo, S. P. (2010). The use of speech generating devices in communication interventions for individuals with developmental disabilities: A review of the literature. *Developmental Neurorehabilitation, 13*, 276–293.

Romski, M. A., & Sevcik, R. A. (1993). Language comprehension: Considerations for augmentative and alternative communication. *Augmentative and Alternative Communication, 9*, 281–285.

Romski, M. A., & Sevcik, R. A. (1996). *Breaking the speech barrier: Language development through augmented means*. Baltimore: Paul H. Brookes Publishing Co.

Romski, M. A., Sevcik, R. A., & Pate, J. L. (1988). Establishment of symbolic communication in persons with severe retardation. *The Journal of Speech and Hearing Disorders, 53*, 94–107.

Russell, T., & Beard, L. (1992). Computer assisted speech as an alternative communication system for the severely multiply handicapped. *The Baylor Educator, 17*, 43–50.

Schepis, M. M., & Reid, D. H. (1995). Effects of a voice output communication on interactions between support personnel and an individual with multiple disabilities. *Journal of Applied Behavior Analysis, 28*, 73–77.

Schepis, M. M., Reid, D. H., & Behrman, M. M. (1996). Acquisition and functional use of voice output communication by persons with profound multiple disabilities. *Behavior Modification, 20*, 451–468.

Schepis, M. M., Reid, D. H., Behrman, M. M., & Sutton, K. A. (1998). Increasing communicative interactions of young children with autism using a voice output communication aid and naturalistic teaching. *Journal of Applied Behavior Analysis, 31*, 561–578.

Schlosser, R. W., & Blischak, D. M. (2001). Is there a role for speech output in interventions for persons with autism? A review. *Focus on Autism and Other Developmental Disabilities, 16*, 170–178.

Schlosser, R. W., Sigafoos, J., & Koul, R. K. (2009). Speech output and speech-generating devices in autism spectrum disorders. In P. Mirenda & T. Iacono (Eds.), *Autism spectrum disorders and AAC* (pp. 141–169). Baltimore: Paul H. Brookes Publishing Co.

Schweigert, P. (1989). Use of microswitch technology to facilitate social contingency awareness as a basis for early communication skills. *Augmentative and Alternative Communication, 5*, 192–198.

Sigafoos, J., & Drasgow, E. (2001). Conditional use of aided and unaided AAC: A review and clinical case demonstration. *Focus on Autism and Other Developmental Disabilities, 16*, 152–161.

Sigafoos, J., & Iacono, T. (1993). Selecting augmentative communication devices for persons with severe disabilities: Some factors for educational teams to consider. *Australia and New Zealand Journal of Developmental Disabilities, 18*, 133–146.

Sigafoos, J., & Roberts-Pennell, D. (1999). Wrong-item format: A promising intervention for teaching socially appropriate forms of rejecting to children with developmental disabilities? *Augmentative and Alternative Communication, 15*, 135–140.

Sigafoos, J., Pennell, D., & Versluis, J. (1996). Naturalistic assessment leading to effective treatment of self-injury in a young boy with multiple disabilities. *Educational and Treatment of Children, 19*, 101–123.

Sigafoos, J., O'Reilly, M. F., Drasgow, E., & Reichle, J. (2002). Strategies to achieve socially acceptable escape and avoidance. In J. Reichle, D. R. Beukelman, & J. C. Light (Eds.), *Exemplary practices for beginning communicators: Implications for AAC* (pp. 157–186). Baltimore: Paul H. Brookes.

Sigafoos, J., Drasgow, E., Halle, J. W., O'Reilly, M. F., Seely-York, S., Edrisinha, C., & Andrews, A. (2004a). Teaching VOCA use as a communicative repair strategy. *Journal of Autism and Developmental Disorders, 34*, 411–422.

Sigafoos, J., Drasgow, E., Reichle, J., O'Reilly, M., Green, V. A., & Tait, K. (2004b). Tutorial: Teaching communicative rejecting to children with severe disabilities. *American Journal of Speech-Language Pathology, 13*, 31–42.

Sigafoos, J., O'Reilly, M. F., Seely-York, S., Weru, J., Son, S., Green, V. A., & Lancioni, G. E. (2004c). Transferring AAC intervention to the home. *Disability and Rehabilitation, 26*, 1330–1334.

Sigafoos, J., O'Reilly, M. F., Ganz, J. B., Lancioni, G. E., & Schlosser, R. W. (2005). Supporting self-determination in AAC interventions by assessing preference for communication devices. *Technology and Disability, 17*, 143–153.

Sigafoos, J., Ganz, J., O'Reilly, M., & Lancioni, G. (2008). Evidence-based practice in the classroom: Evaluating a procedure for reducing perseverative requesting in an adolescent with autism and severe intellectual disability. *Australasian Journal of Special Education, 32*, 55–65.

Sigafoos, J., O'Reilly, M. F., & Lancioni, G. E. (2009). Functional communication training and choice-making interventions for the treatment of problem behavior in individuals with autism spectrum disorders. In P. Mirenda & T. Iacono (Eds.), *Autism spectrum disorders and AAC* (pp. 333–353). Baltimore: Paul H. Brookes Publishing Co.

Sigafoos, J., Arthur-Kelly, M., & Butterfield, N. (2006). *Enhancing everyday communication in children with disabilities*. Baltimore: Paul H. Brookes Publishing Co.

Sigafoos, J., Wermink, H., Didden, R., Green, V. A., Schlosser, R. W., O'Reilly, M. F., & Lancioni, G. E. (2011). Effects of varying lengths of synthetic speech output on augmented requesting and natural speech production in an adolescent with Klinefelter syndrome. *Augmentative and Alternative Communication, 27*, 163–171.

Snell, M. E., & Brown, F. (2006). *Instruction of students with severe disabilities* (6th ed.). Upper Saddle River: Pearson.

Sobsey, D., & Reichle, J. (1989). Components of reinforcement for attention signal switch activation. *Mental Retardation and Learning Disabilities Bulletin, 17*, 46–59.

Soto, G., Belfiore, P. J., Schlosser, R. W., & Haynes, C. (1993). Teaching specific requests: A comparative analysis of skill acquisition and preference using two augmentative and alternative communication aids. *Education and Training in Mental Retardation, 28*, 169–178.

Spiegel, B. B., Benjamin, B. J., & Spiegel, S. A. (1993). One method to increase spontaneous use of an assistive communication device: Case study. *Augmentative andAlternative Communication, 9*, 111–118.

Sutherland, D., Sigafoos, J., Schlosser, R. W., O'Reilly, M. F., & Lancioni, G. E. (2010). Are speech-generating devices viable AAC options for adults with intellectual disabilities? In J. Mullennix & S. Stern (Eds.), *Computer synthesized speech technologies: Tools for aiding impairment* (pp. 161–176). Hershey: Medical Information Science Reference.

Thunberg, G., Ahlsen, E., & Sandberg, A. (2009a). Interaction and use of speech-generating devices in the homes of children with autism spectrum disorders – An analysis of conversational topics. *Journal of Special Education Technology, 24*, 1–17.

Thunberg, G., Sandberg, A., & Ahlsen, E. (2009b). Speech-generating devices used at home by children with autism spectrum disorders: A preliminary assessment. *Focus on Autism and Other Developmental Disabilities, 24*, 104–115.

Trembath, D., Balandin, S., Togher, L., & Stancliffe, R. J. (2009). Peer-mediate teaching and augmentative and alternative communication for preschool-aged children with autism. *Journal of Intellectual and Developmental Disability, 34*, 173–186.

Trottier, N., Kamp, L., & Mirenda, P. (2011). Effects of peer-mediated instruction to teach use of speech-generating devices to students with autism in social games routines. *Augmentative and Alternative Communication, 27*, 26–39.

Van Acker, R., & Grant, S. H. (1995). An effective computer-based requesting system for persons with Rett syndrome. *Journal of Childhood Communication Disorders, 16*, 31–38.

van der Meer, L., & Rispoli, M. J. (2010). Communication interventions involving speech-generating devices for children with autism: A review of the literature. *Developmental Neurorehabilitation, 13*, 294–306.

van der Meer, L., Sigafoos, J., O'Reilly, M. F., & Lancioni, G. E. (2011a). Assessing preferences for AAC options in communication interventions for individuals with developmental disabilities: A review of the literature. *Research in Developmental Disabilities, 32*, 1422–1431.

van der Meer, L., Kagohara, D., Achmadi, D., Green, V. A., Herrington, C., Sigafoos, J., et al. (2011b). Teaching functional use of an iPodbased speech-generating device to individuals with developmental disabilities. *Journal of Special Education Technology, 26*, 1–11.

Wacker, D. P., Wiggins, B., Fowler, M., & Berg, W. K. (1988). Training students with profound or multiple handicaps to make requests via microswitches. *Journal of Applied Behavior Analysis, 21*, 331–343.

White, A. R., Carney, E., & Reichle, J. (2010). Group-item and directed scanning: Examining preschoolers' accuracy and efficiency in two augmentative communication symbol selection methods. *American Journal of Speech-Language Pathology, 19*, 311–320.

Chapter 4
Instructional Technology for Promoting Writing, Work, and Leisure Skills

Abstract This chapter provides an overview of studies assessing the use of technology to enable individuals with severe/profound and multiple disabilities to learn to write, engage in occupational and vocational activities, and access leisure activities. The first part of this chapter analyzes studies that used technology solutions to enable writing by individuals who could not use standard implements such as pens and standard computer keyboards because of their multiple disabilities. The second part of this chapter analyzes studies that used technology to teach individuals to engage in occupational and vocational tasks. These studies used a variety of technology aids as instruction cues, including picture prompts, object or tactile prompts, self-operated audio prompts, self-instruction prompts, video modeling and video prompts, palmtop-based job aids, and electronic control devices. The third part of this chapter analyzes studies on leisure skills that used technology to provide individuals access to different classes of leisure activities, that is, technology that enabled them to access a variety of preferred stimulation and taught them to operate standard or adapted leisure modalities (e.g., radio, television, portable media player, and a computer for e-mail) and an electronic messaging system. The final part of this chapter summarizes the overall outcomes, discusses practical aspects of using technology, and briefly highlights areas for further research in each of these areas.

Introduction

Individuals with severe/profound and multiple disabilities are at great risk for being the passive recipient of services rather than being actively involved in their own well-being. The benevolent intentions of caregivers, including parents, are often at odds with the philosophy of self-determination, which advocates that instruction in the component elements of self-determined behavior be incorporated into existing interventions for all individuals with disabilities (Wehmeyer et al. 2007). The component elements of self-determination include goal setting and attainment, choice

G.E. Lancioni et al., *Assistive Technology: Interventions for Individuals with Severe/Profound and Multiple Disabilities*, Autism and Child Psychopathology Series, DOI 10.1007/978-1-4614-4229-5_4,

making, problem solving, decision making, self-regulation and self-directed learning, self-advocacy, perceptions of efficacy and control, and self-awareness and self-knowledge (Wehmeyer and Field 2007). Given the extensive range of disabilities evidenced in individuals with severe/profound and multiple disabilities, as well as the traditional acceptance of low caregiver expectations, traditional instructional methods have not considered including many component elements of self-determination.

Self-management is one component of self-determination that has received recent attention, particularly with technology-based instruction. There is little support in the research literature for the effectiveness of many traditional methods of instruction for individuals who function in the severe and profound range of intellectual disabilities. Typically, caregivers and teachers have assumed that the diminished cognitive capacity of these individuals preempted them from learning new skills rather than assuming that we must find instructional technology that matches the individuals' needs.

Assistive technology has provided a viable modality to teach a variety of skills, including academic, occupational and vocational skills, and leisure skills. The focus of academic skills has largely been on writing, and we review several studies in which the authors developed innovative assistive technology that enabled the participants to engage in written communication. A range of low-tech prompts have been used with traditional instruction techniques to enable the mastery of various occupation and vocational skills, as well as a few high-tech prompts for those with whom no other techniques had worked previously. However, with leisure activities, there has been an enormous growth in terms of assistive technology, and there is a plethora of studies showing how technology can be customized to meet the needs of individuals regardless of their extensive multiple disabilities.

This chapter provides an overview of studies assessing the use of technology to enable individuals with severe/profound and multiple disabilities to learn to write, engage in occupational and vocational activities, and access leisure activities. The first part of this chapter analyzes studies that developed new technology solutions to enable writing by individuals who could not use traditional implements such as pens and standard computer keyboards because of their multiple disabilities. The second part of this chapter analyzes studies that used technology to teach individuals to engage in occupational and vocational tasks. These studies used a variety of technology aids as instruction cues, including picture prompts, object or tactile prompts, self-operated audio prompts, self-instruction prompts, video modeling and video prompts, palmtop-based job aids, and electronic control devices. The third part of this chapter analyzes studies on leisure skills that used technology to provide individuals access to different classes of leisure activities, that is, technology that enabled them to access a variety of preferred stimulation and taught them to operate standard or adapted leisure modalities (e.g., radio, television, portable media players, and a computer for e-mail) and to use an electronic messaging system. The final part of this chapter summarizes the overall outcomes, discusses practical aspects of using technology, and briefly highlights areas for further research in each of these areas.

Studies on Academic Instruction: Writing

Writing is a basic academic skill that all children learn in early childhood education. The skills involved can be somewhat complex for children in regular education, but more so for those with intellectual and/or physical disabilities. The situation is compounded for those with severe multiple disabilities because their motor deficits may hinder use of either pens or pencils effectively. This can be ameliorated to some extent through the use of technology, especially computers.

If an individual with severe disabilities is able to use a standard computer keyboard, writing can be made more efficient by utilizing a word-processing program that includes word prediction (Williams 2002). While it has its advantages, it does pose some problems as well. For example, because the list of predicted words appear on the screen as the student progresses through writing, attending to and making choices from this list of words may constitute a visual-cognitive burden for students, especially for those with serious/profound and multiple disabilities (Tam et al. 2002). This burden can be lessened by using software with word prediction function that (a) works on a relatively restricted number of words, (b) avoids the use of a screen window with lists of predicted words, and (c) provides a full word in letters and speech when there is high confidence that such a word is the correct one (Barnard and Johnson 2005).

For example, Antonucci et al. (2006) described a study in which they used a writing program with a modified word prediction function. The participant was a 20-year-old man who had severe spastic tetraparesis and multiple disabilities, including being confined to a wheelchair and no speech, but he could emit various types of vocalizations that could be contextually interpreted only by those familiar with him. However, he could use a word-processing system combined with a special keyboard and speech synthesizer. He used roughly 300 different words to write a large variety of sentences dealing with regular daily events, familiar people, activities, and stories. Writing was his basic means of clear communication, supplemented by his vocalizations. His problem with the writing process was that it was very slow and excessively time consuming.

Antonucci et al. (2006) developed and used a word-prediction software in this study that (a) avoided the appearance of a window with predicted words on the computer screen and (b) completed and spoke the word the man was writing when there was certainty that such a word was the one he aimed at within the adopted vocabulary. Typically, the word was completed and spoken after the man had typed its third letter. This was made possible because only a 400-word vocabulary of the words the man most frequently used in his writing was adopted. Using an ABAB reversal design (Barlow et al. 2009), the authors showed that the man's writing equivalent sentences with the word prediction software was much faster than without it. Anecdotal staff data indicated the man's clear preference for the word prediction software. Furthermore, social validation data showed that 40 independent raters scored the word prediction software as significantly more effective than the word-processing program without word prediction.

The situation for an individual who cannot use a standard keyboard for typing because of multiple physical disabilities presents a completely different set of problems (Turpin et al. 2005). Such an individual may find a pointing device, such as a computer mouse or trackball, difficult to operate because of uncoordinated fine hand and finger movements and impaired hand-eye coordination skills (Brodwin et al. 2004). Typical problems involved in using a standard mouse include an inability to correctly aim at small targets on the computer screen and difficulty in actually moving a mouse or in controlling the buttons on the mouse (e.g., an inability to press the buttons or to move the cursor before clicking). Researchers have developed various prototypic hardware and software to enable such an individual access to a computer. For example, Evans et al. (2000) developed a head-operated joystick using infrared light-emitting diodes and photodetectors to determine head position, which subsequently converted into mouse signals. Chen (2001) developed a head-operated computer mouse that included two tilt sensors mounted on a headset that monitored the direction of the person's head up, down, left, and right, and moved the cursor accordingly. Other, more elaborate systems include a "computer mouse" which tracks the individual's movements, including but not restricted to head movements, with a video camera and translates the movements into corresponding movements of the cursor on the computer screen (Betke et al. 2002). While useful, these adaptations have various disadvantages due to their specific design in terms of generalizability, much higher cost when compared to standard devices, can be difficult to obtain and maintain than standard devices, and may not be suitable for some individuals who cannot use head or body movements to control the cursor. Thus, simpler and economical technological solutions are warranted.

Lancioni et al. (2007b) provide an example of a simple and cost-effective approach to using technology that enabled two people with pervasive developmental disabilities to write via a scanning keyboard emulator. The first study involved a young man of 18 years who had severe spastic tetraparesis with very serious problems of spastic hypertonia. He had no functional movement of arms, hands, legs, and trunk. He was able to speak but his speech was difficult to understand and very difficult for him to produce due to prior tracheotomy. He could understand spoken language as well as written text. He could not use standard computer programs due to laborious and unclear speech, inability to use body movements, and difficult control of minimal head turning movements. The authors custom-designed an optic sensor (i.e., a special microswitch; see also Chap. 2) and used a commercial scanning keyboard emulator, together with a portable personal computer. The optic sensor was a light-dependent resistor held through a wire in front of his mouth. He could activate this sensor by covering the light-dependent area by protruding his tongue. The scanning keyboard emulator was adapted to his specific needs by reducing the number of keys used and the key scanning speed. Results showed that when compared to baseline levels, the mean time required for writing each letter of words presented to him decreased, and the total number of letters and words written per session increased dramatically with the introduction of the technology aids.

The second study involved a young lady of 19 years who had severe spastic tetraparesis with very serious problems of spastic hypertonia due to premature birth and perinatal hypoxia. She had no expressive language, but she could understand spoken language as well as written text. She used slight head or eye movements to indicate "yes" and "no." It was difficult for her to use a computer because of lack of motor control except for minimal finger movement. The authors used an optic sensor for an eyelid response (see Lancioni et al. 2006) and a commercial scanning keyboard emulator, together with a portable personal computer. The optic sensor was mounted on the frame of an eyeglass and consisted of a light-emitting diode and an infrared light-detection device. She could activate the sensor by turning her eyes to the right. Results showed an almost 80 % reduction in mean time required to write letters and an increase in the number of letters and words written during a session. In both studies, preference checks showed that both participants preferred the optic sensors and related tongue and eye responses to the pressure or tilt devices and related head and finger responses available to them before this study. Furthermore, social validation ratings by teacher trainees and psychology students showed the new technology was much more highly favored than the old.

Lancioni et al. (2009) described a study in which they assessed the utility of a vocal-detecting sensor and a scanning keyboard emulator for writing. The vocal-detecting sensor was used instead of the optic sensors and tongue- and eye-movement responses because the participants had control of their vocalizations. The voice-detecting sensor consisted of a battery-powered electronic unit, which was linked to a throat microphone and an airborne microphone. The sensors could be activated by a brief vocal emission that triggered both microphones.

The participants were two boys who were using a combination of pressure sensor and scanning keyboard emulator for writing, but they were not comfortable with the head or hand response required for activating the pressure sensor. The boys were almost 13 and 11 years old and had severe spastic tetraparesis due to perinatal hypoxia. Both used wheelchairs and displayed only limited movements of arms, hands, legs, and trunk. They could understand spoken language as well as basic written text. Results showed that the mean time required to write letters using the voice-detecting sensor together with the scanning keyboard emulator was about the same as when they used the pressure sensors. However, preference checks showed that the boys much preferred the voice-detecting sensor to the pressure sensors. Furthermore, social validation ratings by psychology students were significantly higher for the voice-detecting sensor than the ratings for the pressure sensors.

Lancioni et al. (2010a) extended the findings of the previous studies by including participants with responses and microswitches different from those previously used to account for heterogeneity of people with severe/profound and multiple disabilities. Of the two participants in Study 1, the first was a 22-year-old man who was in a wheelchair and had serious problems with fine motor coordination due to degenerative ataxia. He lacked self-help skills, he could not write through standard or adapted keyboards, and his verbal articulation problems made his verbal communication difficult to understand. He used a technology-based writing program at home that consisted of a pressure sensor fixed to the tabletop and connected to a scanning keyboard emulator. He could activate the sensor by making a pushing response produced through a downward movement of his hand. This movement was cumbersome and frustrating for him to make because of his very limited coordination. The second participant was a 9-year-old boy with severe cerebral palsy with spastic tetraparesis and very serious problems of hypertonia with multiple dystonic movements. He was in a wheelchair and had no functional responses of arms, hands, legs, and trunk. He had no expressive language but could understand spoken language as well as written words. He used the same technology-based writing program as the other participant and had similar issues with it.

The new technology used in this study consisted of a small touch/pressure panel serving as a microswitch for a hand response that was considered fairly undemanding when compared to the one previously used by these participants, and a commercial scanning keyboard emulator, with a portable personal computer. The touch/pressure panel was affixed to the table that the participants used during the experimental sessions, in front (man) or to the right (boy) of them. The man activated the touch/pressure panel by a small sliding movement of his hands forward, and the boy activated it by a small sliding movement of his right hand to the right side. The scanning keyboard emulator was adapted in terms of the number of keys used and key scanning speed to match the participants' abilities. Results showed that not only did the participants prefer to use the new touch/pressure panels, but the time they took to write letters was much shorter when compared to their use of the old technology. Indeed, the data showed decreasing time required to type letters with increasing use of the new technology.

The participant in Study 2 was a 12-year-old girl with gross and fine motor disabilities due to mitochondrial leukoencephalopathy, who could ambulate with a walker but required assistance with self-care activities. Although her school had provided her with an expanded keyboard because of her serious problems with writing, she found it frustrating and tiresome to use. The new technology used with her consisted of a small touch/pressure panel and a voice-detecting device that served as microswitches for a hand response and vocalization, and a commercial scanning keyboard emulator, with a portable personal computer. Results showed that although the time taken to write single letters of words was about the same for both the old (expanded keyboard) and new technologies, the participant clearly preferred the new technology. Furthermore, social validation assessment by university psychology students showed much higher ratings for the new over the old technology.

In a further extension of this line of enhancing technology to facilitate writing by persons with severe/profound and multiple disabilities, Lancioni et al. (2011g) developed customized microswitches for three participants in this study. The participants were 13, 45, and 46 years old. The first participant had severe cerebral palsy with spastic tetraparesis and very serious problems of hypertonia with multiple dystonic movements. She was in a wheelchair and had no specific functional responses. She could speak with extreme difficulty and could be understood only by immediate family members, but she could understand spoken language and written text. She used a computer-supported keyboard that could be used through a modified joystick sensor. The second participant had minimal motor abilities and adaptive behavior due to spastic tetraparesis with dystonic movements. He was in a wheelchair, he spoke with some difficulty, but his words were not clear to listeners.

He had tried technological approaches to help him write, including a pressure microswitch for a foot response to operate a scanning keyboard emulator that he found very tiring. Furthermore, using a voice-detecting microswitch relying on an airborne microphone for vocal emissions was found to be unreliable. The third participant had spastic tetraparesis and epilepsy and was confined to a wheelchair. His physical condition was similar to that of the second participant. He used a keyboard with keyguard cover for his writing program, but he found it to be very tiring and thus used it only for brief periods.

Customized microswitches were developed for the three participants. For the first participant, it consisted of a touch/pressure device attached to the palm of her right hand that she could activate with a small hand-closure response. For the second participant, it consisted of a voice-detecting device, with airborne and throat microphones that prevented false microswitch activations due to environmental noise or dystonic movements. For the third participant, it consisted of a touch pad fixed on his right leg, which he could activate by stroking his right hand that he normally rested on that leg. The participants also used a commercially available keyboard emulator, with a portable personal computer, that was adjusted to their needs in terms of the number of keys used and the key spanning speed. Results showed that all three participants preferred their customized microswitches and decreased the writing time per letter for two of the three participants. For the third participant, it was clear that he considered the touch/pressure microswitch and small hand stroking response with the scanning keyboard emulator to be easy and comfortable, and did not show any signs of tiredness, while he found the use of the keyboard with the keyguard cover to be physically demanding and tiring.

In a final study, Lancioni et al. (2011c) extended the use of computer technology for writing to a man who emerged from a minimally conscious state. The man was 47 years old and had a diagnosis of multiple disabilities (neuromotor, consciousness, and communication) following cerebral aneurysm rupture and coma. He had spastic tetraparesis and minimal head control, lacked trunk and sphincteric control, and needed tracheostomy and gastrostomy tube. His wife used a communication board with him that he could activate with a pointing device connected to the middle finger of his right hand (i.e., the only hand that he could partially move). A custom-built programmable computer-aided system, with specific letter presentation and writing functions, was developed for him. When compared to the communication board, the computer-aided system proved more effective in helping the man to engage in clear and readable writing. His new writing prowess enabled him to achieve better communication with his caregivers and family members.

In summary, these studies showed that individuals with severe/profound and multiple disabilities could be assisted to engage effectively in an academic activity like writing to enhance their communication with caregivers, family, and friends. While there are no studies using traditional handwriting methods with this population (Joseph and Konrad 2009), writing can be enabled through the use of technology, thereby enhancing the quality of their lives through communication with a wider community of people.

Studies on Work-Related Outcomes

Individuals with severe/profound and multiple disabilities could acquire increasing independence if they can be taught skills that may give them access to important life domains, such as self-care, literacy, transportation, and work. Technology is increasingly used to improve their work outcomes by enhancing their strengths, maximizing their current potential, and by customizing methods for job skill development. Both low-tech (e.g., picture cards, audio and visual prompts) and high-tech methods (e.g., computer-aided systems) have been used to provide vocational supports to individuals with severe/profound or multiple disabilities (Wehmeyer et al. 2006). Even with people with severe/profound disabilities, the vision is that with appropriate assistance individuals can be taught to acquire and maintain constructive occupation with optimum levels of supervision (Brown et al. 1979). Indeed, there are examples in the research literature of individuals with severe disabilities learning remunerative vocational skills, such as janitorial skills (Cuvo et al. 1978) and various assembly tasks (Horner and McDonald 1982; Hunter and Bellamy 1976).

The early studies relied heavily on low-tech self-management strategies such as picture prompts, object or tactile prompts, self-operated audio prompts, self-instruction prompts, and video modeling and video prompts (Lancioni and O'Reilly 2001). The more recent studies have relied on computer-aided systems, such as using palmtop computers, and other electronic control devices to assist individuals to gain prevocational or occupational skills.

Self-management of Instruction Cues

Picture Prompts

Picture prompts have been used to teach a number of skills to individuals with severe/profound and multiple disabilities. This technique involves training the participants to use photographs or line drawings of successive steps of a task analysis to help them complete a given task. This technique has been used to teach a variety of work skills to individuals with severe disabilities, including vocational tasks (e.g., Wacker and Berg 1983), manage work and break time (Sowers et al. 1980), independently change work tasks (Connis 1979), and initiate a series of vocational tasks (Sowers et al. 1985).

For example, Wacker and Berg (1984) taught three adolescents who functioned in the moderate to severe range of intellectual disabilities to set up workstations independently using picture prompts. They used two tasks: valve assembly, and packaging and setup. The picture prompts consisted of black-and-white photographs of how to set up the valve assembly task and similar pictures of the parts and cards containing colored horizontal lines for the packaging and setup. The pictures were sequenced and bound into a book that the individuals could use as prompts to complete the two tasks. Using a multiple baseline (across both subjects and tasks) with reversal design (Barlow et al. 2009), Wacker and Berg (1984) demonstrated that following just four training sessions, the adolescents could complete the valve assembly task errorlessly. Similar results were obtained with the packaging and setup task, which was used to assess generalization of skills learned with the first task. This study demonstrated that not only could the adolescents rapidly learn the occupational skill through picture prompts, but they also generalize the skills to a second task.

In a follow-up study, Wacker et al. (1985) taught three adolescents who functioned in the severe to profound range of intellectual disabilities to use picture prompts to complete three complex vocational or daily living tasks. The adolescents were taught to complete one task each, and following training, their performance was assessed on two generalization tasks. For example, one of the adolescents learned to dust tables in an apartment, and his generalization tasks were (a) to clean a window and (b) to complete a 22-step conduit-assembly task. Results showed that although the adolescents required extensive training on the initial task, they were able to generalize their use of picture prompts across settings and required substantially reduced amounts of training on the generalization tasks. Furthermore, during maintenance, two adolescents were able to maintain high levels of accurate performance with and without the use of picture prompts, while the third continued to need picture prompts.

Wilson et al. (1987) taught a 36-year-old man with severe intellectual disabilities to use picture prompts to perform a variety of food service tasks at a restaurant. He had good receptive language skills, but poor expressive language. He communicated with a combination of gestures and some vocalizations, which could be understood only by those who knew him well. He was taught four task-analyzed skills: packaging silverware, packing hot sauce, packaging sour cream, and dishwashing. Picture prompts were used to teach all four tasks within a multiple probe design. Results showed that he was able to learn and independently perform all four skills, maintain those skills, and continue to impress his employers with his correct performance 20 months following the termination of training.

Singh et al. (1995) taught three adults who functioned in the profound range of intellectual disabilities to cook using a commercial picture prompt cookbook. Each adult was taught to make a dessert that involved 16 sequenced steps. Following baseline, the three adults engaged in five rehearsal sessions in which they repeated the task steps modeled by the trainers. This was followed by training in cooking with the pictorial instructions. The trainers used error correction and social reinforcement to enhance training outcomes. All three adults were able to master the 16-step cooking procedure and maintained their correct task performance over time, as well as generalize their cooking to novel settings.

Anderson et al. (1997) taught three adults, two of whom functioned in the severe range of intellectual disabilities, to use self-arranged picture prompts to increase their engagement with scheduled activities. Engaging in scheduled activities is an important prevocational skill because the kinds of jobs people with severe/profound and multiple disabilities engage in are arranged in sequence, and engaging in them with minimal staff prompts increases their independence and self-esteem. Photographs were taken of the two individuals engaged in a series of activities, and each one then self-arranged the pictures for scheduled activities on a daily basis. When compared to baseline without a schedule, the two adults substantially increased their participation in the scheduled daily activities by using the self-arranged picture prompts.

Object or Tactile Prompts

While picture prompts work well with sighted individuals, they are of little use with those who are blind. One alternative for them is to use objects as prompts, in which objects are used to represent task steps or activities.

Taylor (1987) taught a 21-year-old woman who was deaf, blind, and functioning in the severe range of intellectual disability to prepare three breakfast foods (i.e., cereal, chocolate milk, and juice). She was verbally prompted to use practice cards that contained object cues. Following baseline, she was sequentially taught to prepare cereal, chocolate milk, and juice, respectively. When she learned the first task, that task was moved into maintenance while she learned the second task, and when she learned the second task, the first two tasks were in maintenance while she learned the third task. She took the longest to learn the first task (25 sessions) but dramatically reduced the number of training sessions required for the remaining two (10 and 9 sessions, respectively). This study showed transfer of learning across tasks using object prompts.

Berg and Wacker (1989) taught a 19-year-old woman who was deaf and blind, and functioning in the moderate to severe range of intellectual disabilities to use tactile prompts to learn a vocational task (packaging). They also assessed generalization to variations of this task (i.e., new materials and setting), and the need for continued use of the tactile prompts following training. They used two envelope-stuffing tasks and one bagging task, with one of the envelope-stuffing tasks and the bagging task being used as the generalization tasks. The required materials were placed in separate compartments of a wooden tray. The tactile prompts were either numbers (training set) or letters (generalization set) drawn with glue and covered with sand, with the prompts placed in either numerical or alphabetical order from left to right across compartments. Further, the cues or prompts were attached with Velcro one to a page and bound into a book. The cues in the book were rearranged each session to correspond to the arrangement of the materials to be packaged. Results showed that the woman was able to effectively use the tactile prompts on the training task and generalized her performance to novel tasks and cues. Further, she continued to need the tactile cues to maintain her performance on the tasks. Together with the findings of Taylor (1987), this study suggests that object/tactile prompts function in a manner similar to picture prompts for individuals who are blind and deaf.

Self-operated Audio Prompts

Auditory prompts have been used for two key reasons. First, it is an appropriate medium of instruction for those individuals who are blind and cannot use braille for reading. Second, it provides a method for shifting stimulus control from the teacher/trainer to the individual when self-operated auditory prompts are used. Typically, in a work situation, workers are required to change from one task to the next without assistance from other workers or supervisors. However, people functioning in the severe or profound range of intellectual disabilities may not be able to change tasks or to move from one component of a task to the next without external assistance. In such cases, there are issues related to low productivity rates (Agran et al. 1986), continued dependence on job coaches and limited behavioral maintenance (Rusch 1986), and the likelihood that the individual may engage in off-task behavior while waiting for an externally delivered prompt (Browder and Shapiro 1985). These issues are preempted if workers with severe/profound or multiple disabilities can be taught to self-manage their work prompts.

Self-operated auditory prompts provide a simple self-management option that requires an individual to use an electronic device (e.g., iPod) that has sequenced instructions for initiating and completing a task-analyzed job. The auditory prompts may be guided instructions (i.e., with predetermined pauses between prompts) or instructions to pause or turn off the device while the task steps are being performed. One cautionary note is that given the cognitive limitations of individuals in the severe to profound range of intellectual disabilities, the instructions should be short and easily understood by the participant.

Alberto et al. (1986) taught four adolescents who functioned in the severe range of intellectual disabilities three vocational skills: a vocational assembly task, use of a washing machine, and a food preparation sequence using a self-operated auditory prompting system. They used a Walkman-like tape recorder for the auditory cues. The adolescents wore the recorder on an adjustable belt around the waist and used the accompanying headphones. They used a four-phase experimental sequence, within a multiple baseline design (Barlow et al. 2009) to assess the effects of the self-operated audio prompts: baseline (no prompts), acquisition (recorded prompts with teacher assistance), faded assistance (recorded prompts without teacher assistance), and maintenance (no recorded prompts). Results showed that each of the four adolescents was able to learn with self-operated audio prompts and maintain performance on each task.

Davis et al. (1992) taught three young adults who functioned in the severe range of intellectual disabilities to increase the fluency of their work performance in a community-based food preparation facility. They used a modified stereo cassette player that had the "stop" and "play" buttons color-coded to facilitate independent operation and the fast forward button removed to prevent inadvertent tape movement. Each participant chose a song that they could only play during work, and the instructions (e.g., "Keep working," "Don't stop until the alarm rings") were embedded in the song. These auditory prompts were delivered on a variable time schedule, depending on the intervention phase. Performance fluency was assessed across three conditions within a multiple baseline design: nonmusic baseline, music-only baseline, and self-operated auditory prompts embedded in the music. Results showed all three young adults increased their vocational task fluency when they used the auditory prompts.

These studies, when taken in concert with similar research (e.g., Briggs et al. 1990; Steed and Lutzker 1999), suggest that self-operated audio prompts enable individuals who function in the severe range of intellectual disabilities to learn new vocational skills, to increase the fluency of the existing vocational skills, and to generalize these skills to other tasks and settings.

Self-instruction Prompts

Self-directed verbal prompts have been reported to be effective in enabling individuals with severe intellectual disabilities to learn, maintain, and generalize vocational skills and promote independence (e.g., Agran et al. 1992; Moore et al. 1989; Salend et al. 1989). However, no technology is necessary for teaching verbal self-instruction and thus will not be covered here.

Video Modeling and Video Prompts

Video modeling and video prompting have been used for simulated instruction prior to instruction and performance in another setting. In video modeling, the participants watch a video of a task being performed, discuss the nuances of the task, and then engage in a simulated performance of the task (Lasater and Brady 1995). The participants are then taken to the setting where the task is to be performed, given further instructions, and required to perform the task. In video prompting, the participants are shown a videotape of a model performing each step of the task (LeGrice and Blampied 1994). Instead of seeing the entire videotape, only one video clip is shown at a time, giving the individuals time to perform the first step of the task before seeing the clip for the second step, and so on, until the entire task is completed.

Occasionally, researchers have combined the use of video modeling and video prompts (Martin et al. 1992). These procedures have been found to be effective in teaching vocational skills to individuals who function in the moderate range of intellectual disabilities (Alberto et al. 2005; Cihak et al. 2006a; Goodson et al. 2007). Given previous findings on other forms of prompting, there is no reason why these procedures will not be equally useful in teaching prevocational and vocational skills to individuals who function in the severe range of intellectual disabilities.

Palmtop-Based Job Aid

In an innovate series of studies, Furniss et al. (2001) described the development and evaluation of a palmtop computer that served as a job aid or prompt for individuals who functioned in the severe range of intellectual disabilities. The initial model was based on a Hewlett-Packard HP 2001 × palmtop with an 80C186 central processor, 1 Mb of RAM, and a black-and-white CGA LCD screen. After using and testing the system in the first two studies described below, they enhanced the system by basing it on IBM PC110 palmtop with an Intel 80486SX (33 MHz) central processor; 8 Mb of Ram; a 640×480 DSTN VGA screen (256 colors); infrared, serial, and PCMCIA III communication ports; and the ability to run MS-DOS or Windows operating system. This was paired with a specially designed radio communication system. Both versions provided the individuals with instructional sequences and reminder prompts.

In the first study, Lancioni et al. (1998) assessed the comparative effectiveness of using a palmtop job aid against a card system in the context of occupational task performance of three adults who functioned in the severe range of intellectual disabilities. The three individuals ranged in age from 20 to 32 years, and all attended a day activity center where they were involved in occupational/vocational tasks. For this study, each individual was presented with two tasks (i.e., eight tasks in total). The eight tasks (involving food preparation, cleaning, and table setting) were task-analyzed into 18–32 steps each. The study included five phases: baseline (no prompts), training (use of the palmtop with one task and cards with the other task), maintenance (use of the palmtop with one task and cards with the other task), cross-over (the task that previously employed a palmtop as a prompt now used cards and vice versa), and preference assessment (participants could choose between the two prompt modalities for the next task). When compared to baseline and use of card prompts, correct performance was much higher when palmtop prompts were used. The preference assessment showed that two of the three individuals chose the palmtop over cards.

In the second study, Lancioni et al. (1999b) replicated the previous study with four new participants who also functioned in the severe range of intellectual disability. These individuals were between 18 and 23 years of age, and all attended a day activity center where they engaged in occupational/vocational tasks, such as sorting objects and making embroideries. The procedure used in the first study was essentially replicated with the new participants. Results showed the palmtop system was more effective in terms of task performance with all participants. Furthermore, three of the four participants preferred the palmtop while the fourth preferred the card system.

In the third study, Lancioni et al. (2000) reported two interrelated experiments, both using an enhanced palmtop computer (color screen) and auditory and vibratory prompting mechanisms. This enhanced system was again compared to the card system using different tasks. Six individuals ranging in age from 23 to 47 years and functioning in the severe range of intellectual disabilities participated in Experiment

1. They were chosen because of their reliance on external support to maintain their engagement in simple daily occupations (e.g., putting objects in boxes, painting, and elementary embroideries). Each individual used the palmtop system for one set of tasks and the card system for the other set of tasks in an alternating treatments design (Barlow et al. 2009). The same sequence of experimental phases was used: baseline, training, maintenance, crossover, and preference test. Results showed that the individuals had much higher rates of correct performance with the palmtop system when compared with the card system. Furthermore, when given a choice, the individuals preferred to use the palmtop system on an average of 90 % of the sessions.

Three individuals who performed above 90 % accuracy in the last two phases of Experiment 1 also participated in Experiment 2. The aim was to assess outcome when the number of instructions was reduced and to evaluate whether the new instruction format would maintain satisfactory performance. Instead of being presented individually, about two-thirds of the instructions were either clustered or some instructions were omitted the new instruction format. Results showed the three individuals had 53–61 % correct performance in the noninstruction condition, 73–89 % in the some instructions omitted condition, and 88–97 % in the clustered instructions condition.

In the fourth study, Lancioni et al. (1999a) essentially replicated Experiment 2 from the previous study with four new participants. The four individuals ranged in age from 19 to 39 years, and functioned in the severe range of intellectual disabilities. All attended a day activity center where they engaged in simple occupational/vocational tasks (object assembly, painting, embroidery). They required staff prompts to stay on task because of short attention span. Each individual was taught two tasks, with the palmtop computer presenting one pictorial prompt per task step. Once they mastered the two tasks, the instructions were split into three types: no instructions, some instructions omitted, and instructions clustered. Results showed all four individuals had the most number of correct responses under the clustered instructions condition, followed by some instructions omitted, and no instructions.

In the fifth study, Furniss et al. (1999) assessed the effectiveness of the enhanced palmtop system in real work situations and investigated the views of the participants' caregivers regarding the effectiveness and social acceptability of the palmtop computer prompting system. Six individuals ranging in age from 31 to 47 years and functioning in the severe range of intellectual disabilities participated. All attended day centers and all but one had been excluded from consideration for employment because of the severity of their disabilities. During the study, each individual engaged in work experience, performing a real job in a regular work environment for half a day per week. The first two assembled aqualung pillar valves; the third assembled and packed boxes of catering workers' forage caps; the fourth prepared, stamped, and sorted by department clocking-in cards for the workforce in a general light engineering factory; and the last two assembled and packed kits of nuts, bolts, and washers. Results showed all six individuals were able to use the palmtop prompts effectively by increasing their levels of accurate work performance.

Furthermore, interviews with the participants' caregivers indicated general satisfaction with regard to the overall benefit to the participants.

Other researchers have expanded on the use of palmtop computers to deliver auditory and visual prompts. For example, it has been used to increase performance of functional tasks performed by students with mild to severe intellectual disabilities (Davies et al. 2002a, b, 2003), reduce the amount of time needed to complete tasks and increase the work productivity of students with developmental delays (Riffel et al. 2005), and facilitate generalization across increasingly complex tasks, as well increase the probability of skill maintenance, by adolescents with moderate intellectual disabilities (Cihak et al. 2006b). The palmtop computers used to deliver auditory and verbal prompts are portable and economical devices that can enhance the ability of individuals with severe/profound and multiple disabilities to engage in gainful employment.

Electronic Control Devices

Technology has been used to develop devices that produce visual, auditory, or mechanical (e.g., air blowing) prompts to assist individuals to achieve some degree of independence in their occupation or vocational activities. For example, Lancioni et al. (2011h) presented a case study using a new verbal instruction system to help a woman successfully engage in food- and drink-preparation tasks. She was 31 years old and had congenital encephalopathy linked to polymalformative syndrome, rigidity of the legs due to structural problems of the hips and knees, blindness due to congenital microphthalmia and glaucoma, intellectual disability, and lacked sphincteric control. She attended a day activity center where she engaged in work activities, such as assembling key holders or the bases of baskets. She expressed an interest in the use of verbal-instruction technology to perform food- and drink-preparation tasks. Six food preparation tasks were selected: cold pasta dishes, multiflavor drinks, sandwiches, stuffed breads, yogurt desserts, and blended fruit drinks. These tasks included between 44 and 54 task-analyzed instruction steps.

The verbal instruction system used with her was similar to that used by Lancioni et al. (2010d) for assisting individuals with Alzheimer's disease recover their performance of daily activities. Briefly, it consisted of three radio-frequency photocells, light-reflecting paper, an amplified MP3 player with USB pen drive connection, a pen containing the verbal instructions for the single steps of the task to be performed, and a microprocessor-based electronic control unit. The electronic control unit contained specifically developed software, which allowed it to respond to photocell inputs and to regulate the command functions of the MP3 player and, thus, the presentation of the verbal instructions and the time intervals occurring between them. In the first part of the study, this verbal instruction system was more effective than a control system in enabling the woman to prepare cold pasta dishes and multiflavor drinks. In the second part of the study, she successfully learned to prepare the other four items—sandwiches, stuffed breads, yogurt desserts, and blended fruit drinks. Furthermore, the gains in performance were maintained at an 8-week follow-up. This verbal instruction system enabled the woman to independently engage in an important occupational skill.

Lancioni et al. (2011i) replicated the above study with three adults with multiple disabilities, including visual, physical, intellectual, and medical problems. The three adults ranged in age between 33 and 36 years, suffered from congenital encephalopathy due to infections or complications during pregnancy. They attended care and rehabilitation centers where they were involved in simple occupational and vocational tasks with variable levels of support. The same tasks as in the Lancioni et al. (2010d) study were used, namely, preparation of cold pasta dishes, multiflavor drinks, sandwiches, stuffed breads, yogurt desserts, and blended fruit drinks. Prompts were provided through the new verbal instruction system described in the previous study. The results of this study were in accord with the Lancioni et al. (2010d) study and showed that the new verbal-instruction system was effective in enabling the three individuals to learn and maintain food preparation skills.

In another example of the use of an electronic control device to produce customized automatic prompts, Lancioni et al. (2008b) used air-blowing prompts with two individuals who were deaf and blind, and verbal prompts for another two who were blind but had typical hearing. These prompts were developed to enable the individuals to move through and perform simple occupational activities that were arranged within a room. The four adults ranged in age from 20 to 43 years and were functioning within the profound range of intellectual disability. Three of them were totally blind, and the fourth had minimal residual vision. They attended a center for persons with profound and multiple disabilities that emphasized constructive occupation.

The automatic prompting system consisted of a battery-powered, electronic control device placed at the entrance of the activity room and linked via radio to (a) fan devices placed at the left side of each activity table (for two participants who were both deaf and blind), or voice output boxes at the back of the tables (for the two participants who had hearing) and (b) optic sensors attached to the front edge of the tables. There were eight activity tables, and the individuals had to move from one table to the next to trigger the optic sensor that in turn triggered a programmed prompt, either an air-blowing prompt (from the fans) or a voice prompt at each activity table. Results showed that all four individuals were able to move through and perform the activities at each activity table with the assistance of automatic prompting and independent of staff assistance.

In summary, a number of technological systems have been used to enable people with severe/profound and multiple disabilities to learn and maintain occupational, prevocational, and vocational skills. Not only do these individuals prefer to use technology, especially computer-based systems (Lancioni et al. 2001), but they also develop the ability to engage in socially valued activities that enhance their self-esteem, reduce the probability of them engaging in maladaptive behaviors, enhance social engagement, and increase the likelihood of having a better quality of life.

Studies on Leisure Activities

A common understanding of leisure is that it involves a person choosing and participating in meaningful activity primarily for enjoyment and satisfaction (Dattilo and Schleien 1994). Although leisure has been recognized as an important curricular domain for individuals with severe/profound and multiple disabilities, there is only limited literature on teaching such individuals a range of leisure skills. For example, most individuals who function in the severe to profound range of intellectual disabilities do not learn how to engage in common leisure pursuits (e.g., to independently control a radio or TV, use a computer to send messages, take photographs, use MP3 players or an iPod), and need to be taught such skills (Schleien et al. 1995). Furthermore, although leisure skill training was popular in the research literature for a decade beginning in the late 1970s, there has been a paucity of training and research in this area until recently (Edrisinha et al. 2011). Over the past decade, technology has been used to teach individuals with severe/profound and multiple disabilities a small number of leisure skills. These include the use of microswitches to choose among pleasurable leisure activities and learning to operate radio, TV, multimedia device (iPod), electronic messaging, and computer for e-mails.

Microswitches

Individuals with severe/profound and multiple disabilities are often unable to interact with standard leisure equipment because of their extensive neuromotor and sensory deficits. If left on their own, they become isolated and slowly lose whatever skills they may possess through lack of constructive engagement with their environment. This then precludes self-determination in terms of their leisure time because they are presented with leisure activities chosen by their caregivers at prescheduled times that are convenient for staff or family members (Algozzine et al. 2001). Thus, they become recipients of external input rather than active agents who can pick and choose what activities to engage in and when they wish to engage in them.

Microswitches have been used to customize technology that enables people with severe/profound and multiple disabilities to make choices and interact with their environment (Lancioni et al. 2005a, 2011f). This technology overcomes many of the issues prevalent with standard leisure products and processes. Thus, microswitches can be used to control environmental events with simple responses, often with minimal effort (Crawford and Schuster 1993; Mechling 2006). The neat thing about microswitches is that they can be customized to whatever large or small movement the individual still possesses and uses that movement to activate a large number of activities (Lancioni et al. 2011d; Varona et al. 2008). For example, if at all a person can control is eye blinking, then an optic microswitch fixed to the frame of an eyeglass and connected to a timer and an MP3 player may enable the individual to listen to music through repeated eyelid closure.

A plethora of studies have been undertaken with a large number of microswitches that enable individuals with severe/profound and multiple disabilities to access stimulation, including songs, music, games, stories, familiar voices, television, family members, friends, vibrotactile events, massagers, flickering lights, light fiber compositions, light tubes with bubbling effects, alarm sounds, doorbell sounds, voices of family members, light air puff, and so on. In all of these studies, the participants learned to use customized microswitches to access brief periods of stimulation (e.g., Lancioni et al. 2004, 2005a, 2006, 2007c, 2011a; Tota et al. 2006).

In the above studies, the individuals accessed brief periods of stimulation from an array provided by the software (see also Chap. 2). In the studies discussed below, the individuals actively engaged with a leisure modality and made their own choices in terms of when to access the leisure activity and for how long.

Radio

Managing to use a radio opens a major leisure modality for an individual who is virtually immobile and permanently confined to bed. Self-directed use of a radio enables the individual to be in touch with daily news, music, plays, politics, and specialty programs, among others.

Lancioni et al. (2011e) reported two studies, one of which involved providing technological assistance to a man so that he could use a radio. The man was 52 years of age and confined to a totally static supine position in bed due to multiple sclerosis. He had a permanent tracheostomy tube and received mechanical ventilation. His voluntary motor responses were reduced to minimal movements of his chin to the left, small movements of the lips, and eye closures. Given his precarious medical condition, he lived in a medical care center under close supervision. He enjoyed the company of family members and caregivers and liked to listen to the radio.

The technology assistance included a modified radio digital device, a microprocessor-based electronic control unit, a microswitch, an amplified MP3 player with USB pen drive connection, a pen containing verbal questions on radio operations (i.e., to change programs and switching the radio on and off), and two different earpieces connected to the radio and MP3 player, respectively. When all of the technology aids were hooked up, the microprocessor-based electronic unit served to present to the man choices that he could make (i.e., choice of radio programs or to switch off the radio) via a microswitch that he could activate by a slight movement of his chin, and to carry out his choices. Results showed that following training with the new technology, the man was able to self-initiate radio programs that he wanted to listen to and also to turn the radio off when he was done. This study showed that an individual who has profound multiple disabilities, including being almost immobile, can be given technological assistance to enhance the quality of his life.

Television

Television is ubiquitous in our society and is often used to inform and entertain us. Like radio, but with visual input, television provides another leisure modality to people who have severe/profound and multiple disabilities. Indeed, it provides all of the benefits of radio plus virtual reality in terms of people, places, and programs. Thus, being able to independently operate a television set would enable individuals to make personal choices with regard to programs they wish to watch, as well as when they would like to watch the programs.

Lancioni et al. (2007a) described a study in which they used technology to assist a young man with multiple disabilities to manage his leisure television engagement independently. He was 18 years old and had severe spastic tetraparesis with very serious problems of spastic hypertonia due to postnatal hypoxia. He had no functional movements of arms, hands, legs, and trunk and was fed via a gastrostomy tube. His speech was difficult to understand and laborious to produce. He lay in bed with the body and face rotated to his right. The aim of the study was to help him to independently turn the television on and off, select a channel, and increase or decrease the volume.

The technology involved three microswitches, an electronic control system, and a television remote-control device. The first microswitch was a pressure device placed on the right side of the young man's face and served to select one of the three sequenced functions built within the electronic control system, that is, on/off, channels, and volume control. Each activation of the microswitch, which was produced by a slight movement of his face to the right, resulted in the selection of the next function in this arrangement. The other two microswitches were optic sensors (which could be activated by a protrusion of the tongue) placed at the left and right sides of his lower lip. They enabled the television-management responses via the electronic control system and the remote-control device. For example, if the on/off function was selected via the first microswitch, activation of the left sensor turned off the television, while activation of the right sensor turned it on. If the channel function was selected, activation of the left sensor led to previous channels in the sequence, while activation of the right sensor led to subsequent channels in the sequence. Finally, if the volume function was selected, activation of the left sensor decreased the volume, while activation of the right sensor increased it. Results showed that the technology helped this young man to operate his television without caregiver assistance. Preference assessment showed that he preferred to be independent in managing his leisure television. Furthermore, 90 teacher trainees provided social validation of the new technology by rating it very positively.

Lancioni et al. (2010b) described a technology-based program that promoted independent television use by a man with acquired brain injury and multiple disabilities. The man was 46 years old and had neuromotor, consciousness, and communication disabilities following cerebral aneurysm rupture and coma. He had tetraparesis, lack of trunk control, minimal head control, epilepsy, an absence of sphincteric control, and used gastrostomy tube for enteral nutrition. He had previous experience with microswitches, but he wanted to watch television programs without assistance from his caregivers.

The technology involved two microswitches, a microprocessor-based electronic control unit, an amplified MP3 player with USB pen drive connection, a pen containing the recording of verbal instructions (i.e., information statements concerning television operations and responses), and an adapted remote-control device. The first microswitch was a pressure-sensitive device placed on the man's wheelchair tray.

Its activation signaled to the electronic control unit to activate the MP3 player, which emitted a verbal instruction about a possible operation and the response needed to trigger it. The second microswitch was an optic (photocell) device fixed on his left arm. Activating this microswitch served to confirm the operation indicated in the instruction and to cause the electronic control unit to trigger and execute such an operation. At the start of a session, the verbal instruction was "If you want the television on, touch your arm." Subsequently (i.e., when the man was already watching the television), the instruction would be "If you want to change channel, touch your arm." Touching the arm (i.e., activating the optic device fixed on it) within 8 s from the first instruction led the electronic control unit to switch on the television through the adapted remote-control device. Touching the arm within 8 s from the second instruction led the electronic control unit to change channel. A total of ten channels were programmed, and a change always led to the next one in a circular fashion. Reactivating the pressure-sensitive microswitch after the second instruction led the unit to present (through the MP3 player) the third instruction, which was "If you want the television off, touch your arm." Results showed that the man learned to use his television and could operate it without assistance from family members, thereby becoming more independent and self-sufficient in one leisure activity.

iPod

The iPod is a portable multimedia device, like an MP3 player, that individuals can use to listen to preferred music and watch entertainment videos. It is an age-appropriate skill that provides individuals with severe disabilities a modality for engaging in a preferred leisure activity at times of their choosing.

For example, Kagohara (2011) taught three adolescents, who were 15–19 years old and functioned in the severe range of intellectual disability, to self-operate an iPod Touch® to watch entertainment videos. All three understood simple commands but none of them could carry an age-appropriate conversation. All three attended a public school and were in a class of five students with developmental disabilities. The study was conducted in their classroom. A preference survey indicated the first adolescent enjoyed animation movies, the second enjoyed videos of her classroom and school playground, and the third enjoyed videos of sports such as rugby, soccer, and basketball. Several 30-s video clips aligned with the adolescents' choices were preloaded on their iPods, and new but similar content clips were added as the training progressed to prevent boredom.

A task analysis indicated that inexperienced users can be taught to operate an iPod in seven steps. A 38-s video was made of a person completing the seven steps, and this was used during the video modeling instruction. This video was also uploaded on each adolescent's 16-GB iPod Touch®. The three adolescents were taught how to operate their iPod within a delayed multiple probe across participants design (Barlow et al. 2009), across baseline, video modeling and least-to-most prompting, video fading, and follow-up. Results showed that the three adolescents were able to independently operate their iPods and were able to maintain their correct performance when the video instructions were faded, with follow-up showing 80–100 % accuracy.

In a follow-up study, Kagohara et al. (2011) taught the same three adolescents, who had learned to use the iPod Touch® to watch entertainment videos, to now operate the iPod to listen to music. In the previous study, the contribution of the video modeling and least-to-most prompts to learning outcome could not be separated. Thus, in this study, video modeling alone was used. As in the previous study, a delayed multiple probe across participants design was used across baseline, video modeling, video fading, and follow-up. Video modeling included eight task-analyzed steps for learning how to select and listen to music on the iPod. A 34-s video of the steps being modeled was uploaded on each adolescent's iPod Touch's video list. Results showed that the three adolescents were unable to fully operate the iPod to listen to music during baseline, but they acquired the necessary skills during the video modeling. Furthermore, they were able to maintain their skills when the video modeling was faded and during follow-up.

These two studies demonstrate that individuals who function within the severe range of intellectual disabilities can learn to independently use an iPod Touch® to listen to music and to watch entertainment videos. They also demonstrate that such individuals need not be simply the recipients of leisure activities, but can indeed learn to be self-directed.

E-Mail

E-mails enable an individual to independently communicate with family and friends. For example, Bache and Derwent (2008) presented a case study of a woman in her early 20s with profound disabilities who had sustained a severe head injury following a sports related accident resulting in a large right-sided extradural hematoma leading to a diagnosis of low awareness state. She presented with severe extensor posture of her neck, trunk, pelvis, and upper limbs. With very slow movements, she could turn her head toward the left and slightly across midline to the right, but she had no other voluntary control of any other part of her body. With therapy, a slight movement was noted in her right middle and ring fingers, but she was unable to elicit the movements on command. She was a competent computer user prior to her accident, and electronic communication (i.e., e-mail, text-messaging, and social networking websites) was very important to her.

An initial technology aid provided her with a custom-built touch-sensitive switch that she could activate with her left temple, requiring no force at the end of the rotation. She used this system to write free text messages using an on-screen scanning keyboard. The software required her to scan row-column grids containing letters of the alphabet and punctuation signs. Although this system was slow and laborious, she could write messages. The drawback was that she could not use it for long because the extensor posture in her neck and trunk rapidly fatigued her in this effort. A second technology aid was developed based on her ability to move her eyes up and down quite easily, and horizontally with some effort. Thus, the touch-sensitive switch was replaced by an eye gaze system which enabled her to control the on-screen mouse pointer with her eyes. While there were technical issues that had to be overcome (e.g., she could only scan a part of the computer screen given her limited physical and sensory ability), she was eventually able to use the eye gaze system to write letters and e-mails, and send them to family and friends without assistance from her caregivers. Given that she was physically immobile and had enforced free time, the technology aid gave her a degree of independence in terms of choosing how she would use some of this time.

Enabling individuals with severe/profound and multiple disabilities to use e-mail provides them with opportunities to communicate with distant family, friends, and acquaintances. Furthermore, it has potential therapeutic value in terms of decreasing isolation, reducing the probability of depression, and enhancing self-esteem (Todis et al. 2005). Thus, there has been some emphasis on this form of leisure activity, particularly in individuals with multiple physical and neurological disabilities, such as those with traumatic brain injury (e.g., Egan et al. 2006).

Electronic Messaging

For some individuals, the severity of their multiple disabilities, including extensive motor and visual disabilities, precludes them from using standard or adapted technology for e-mails and telephones (Gartland 2004). For these individuals, technologies need to be customized for their specific disabilities.

Lancioni et al. (2010c) described a study in which they developed a new technology that enabled adults with acquired brain injury and extensive motor, visual, cognitive, and behavioral disabilities to send and receive text messages. The two adults were 39 and 50 years of age. The first adult had suffered an anterolateral myocardial infarction followed by cardiac arrest and postanoxic coma about 6 years prior to the study. At the time of the study, she presented a complex picture of postanoxic encephalopathy with cortical blindness, urinary incontinence, compulsive and occasionally aggressive behavior, rapid frustration, frequent sadness, spastic-dystonic tetraparesis, and spastic dysarthria with slow-labored and difficult-to-understand speech. She could use the telephone but it frustrated her because of her verbal communication problems and her dependence on others for operating it. The second adult had suffered aneurysm rupture at the top of the basilar artery about 7 years prior to the study with consequent surgery and a period of coma for about 3 weeks. At the time of the study, he had minimal visual functioning, anosognosia, urinary incontinence, left hemiparesis with Babinski's signs and severe reduction of any fine motor coordination, apathy, depressive mood, and virtual mutism. He received phone calls from family members, but he hardly responded due to his communication issues.

The technology to send out and receive messages consisted of a netbook computer, a global system for mobile communication (GSM) modem, two microswitches (i.e., an optic device placed at the right ear of the first adult and a pressure device on the wheelchair tray of the second) enabling the participants to activate the computer, an interface connecting the microswitches to the computer, and a specifically developed software program. This program allowed the computer to present information along prearranged schemes, respond to microswitch activations, send out text messages, and read and verbalize incoming messages. The initial microswitch activation triggered the computer to present a list of names to whom the messages could be sent. The only exception occurred if the computer had signaled the presence of unread incoming messages. In that case, microswitch activation led the computer to read those messages. Results showed that, following training, both adults could send and receive messages independently.

Lancioni et al. (2011b) provided further evidence of the utility of the special messaging technology developed for the study described above. In the new study, the two individuals were 54 and 43 years old, both had major injuries due to either a road or work accident (respectively), severe brain injury, and coma following their accidents. Given their extensive physical, motor, and neurocognitive disabilities, both were excellent candidates for using the special messaging technology that was adapted to their unique circumstances.

The effectiveness of the special messaging technology was assessed within a nonconcurrent multiple baseline across participants design (Barlow et al. 2009). Each individual sent and received messages with the help of a research assistant during baseline and without the research assistant during intervention. During intervention, a research assistant provided ten training trials to familiarize both of them with the new technology and the requirements for sending and receiving (listening) messages. During the regular intervention sessions that followed, the computer system reminded the participants of the possibility of sending messages and of the response needed. Results showed that the two individuals could not send or receive messages independent of the research assistant during baseline. During intervention, on average, the two individuals sent more than 85 % and received more than 90 % of the messages independently of the research assistant.

Lancioni et al. (2011e; Study 2) further examined the utility of the special messaging technology with an adolescent who had multiple disabilities. This adolescent was about 17 years old, functioned in the severe range of intellectual disabilities, and had encephalopathy due to perinatal hypoxia and cerebral hemorrhage. He presented with spastic tetraparesis, was in a wheelchair, and was functionally blind. His language was mostly nonintelligible, but he had good receptive language. The effectiveness of the special messaging technology, which had been adapted to his unique abilities, was assessed within a reversal design (Barlow et al. 2009). Results showed he was unable to send or receive messages independently of the research assistant during baseline. Following training on the use of the special messaging system, he was able to send over 90 % of his messages and receive all of his messages independently.

These three studies demonstrate that custom-built messaging technology was effective in enabling leisure communication for individuals for whom no other technology had worked previously. This was possible because the new technology maximized the motoric and cognitive strengths the individuals had. These adaptations enabled these individuals to achieve levels of leisure activity that would be impossible without customized technology. Enabling their capacity for communication also has the added advantage of increased interaction and emotional bonding with family, friends, and acquaintances.

Discussion

Writing

The results reported in the studies on writing were very positive, indicating the individuals were able to use the new technology to their advantage. The new technology used microswitches (sensors) for single, simple responses and scanning keyboard emulators. These sensors were deemed less demanding in terms of physical effort by the individuals when compared to other devices developed for the same purpose that require head movements and cheek puffs or eye rotation and eyelid closures. Overall, the new technology was either as effective or more effective than what had been previously available to the individuals in terms of writing speed, was always less tiring in terms of effort, and was generally preferred by them. Although the total number of participants in these studies was relatively small, there were several successful replications across individuals with different disabilities, suggesting a robust effect of the new technology.

In terms of practical considerations, the microswitches required simple responses such as hand closures, vocalization, hand stroking, tongue protrusion, single eye movement, and finger movements. The use of a keyboard with an automatic scanning function was highly effective with individuals who had extensive motor disabilities. In all likelihood, given their physical limitations, these individuals may well have found it impossible to manage two responses as necessitated by the older technologies, that is, one to move the cursor to the letters required for the target words and the other to select and write those letters (Simpson et al. 2010).

While these studies showed that individuals could reduce the time it took them to write individual letters and words, the absolute times they took was still much higher than those without or with minimal disabilities. Thus, there is still much room to improve the technology (Baker and Moon 2008). For example, the scanning process could be made more functional by reducing the number of keys available and by grouping two or three letters on each of the keys (Lancioni et al. 2011g). Furthermore, combining the visual scanning process with auditory cues from the system may facilitate the identification of the target letters and, eventually, response efficacy. These are issues that future research must answer. An additional research issue concerns social validation of the new technology by the individuals, caregivers, and family members (Callahan et al. 2008).

Developing or enhancing the ability of individuals with extensive motor disabilities to write independently through custom-designed technology is important not only for communicating to caregivers their immediate needs but also to enhance recovery, social networking, and leisure skills. Increasing their writing speed would have beneficial effects beyond just practical considerations because it increases their sense of efficiency and self-efficacy (Anson et al. 2006). Indeed, the use of the writing technology can also be instrumental in enabling them access to electronic mail, Internet, and videogames by combining the microswitches and keyboard emulator with commercial software such as QualiSURF (QualiLife UK, Kent TN15 7DA) (Moisey and Van de Keere 2007).

Occupational and Vocational Skills

The results reported in the studies on occupational and vocational skills were very positive in terms of outcomes of the instructions. The outcomes were measured in terms of learning as opposed to work products. The studies used a number of instructional prompts ranging from low-tech to high-tech solutions. However, regardless of the nature of the prompts used, the individuals were able to master the tasks presented to them (Lancioni and O'Reilly 2001). Of course, the characteristics of the individuals (i.e., severity of cognitive and physical disabilities) varied among the studies, as well as the complexity of the tasks. Simpler instructional prompt techniques appeared to work well with those individuals who had less severe disabilities. Those with severe/profound and multiple disabilities need more customized technological solutions to enable them to learn simple occupational/vocational tasks. Overall, regardless of the nature and/or severity of their disabilities, the individuals were able to acquire the skills they were being taught with the assistive technology they were provided.

Strengths and shortcomings can be identified with each of the instructional techniques. For example, pictures on cards are the most used form of instructional prompts in this population and so ingrained in the system that virtually no recent research has been published on it. It has face validity for teaching a task because it is a simple technique, easy and economical to prepare, and can be easily modified. There are probably only two major drawbacks in using picture prompts. First, they are usually arranged in a book form or stacked in an array, and the individuals need to have the skill to turn the pages or handle the cards one at a time in sequence. These are skills that usually need to be taught to individuals who function in the severe to profound range of intellectual and physical disabilities (Lancioni and Oliva 1988). Thus, a prerequisite for using picture prompts may include systematic training on handling the cards (Wacker et al. 1985). Second, a similar systematic training may be needed with those individuals who have severe cognitive impairments and have not developed an awareness of pictures as representations of objects and actions (Dixon 1981).

Object cues provide an alternative to picture cues and are particularly useful for individuals who have severe visual impairment or blindness. Objects have similar drawbacks as picture prompts. Audio prompts have been used as alternatives to picture and object prompts for individuals with or without visual impairment. Its major shortcoming is that individuals who function in the severe to profound range of intellectual disability usually do not have the necessary receptive language skills to utilize them (Alberto et al. 1986; McLean et al. 1999). A similar problem arises with self-instructional prompts because of the lack of necessary receptive and expressive language capability in individuals with severe or profound intellectual disability to use this self-management strategy (McLean et al. 1999).

Video modeling and video prompts have been used with individuals with mild to moderate intellectual disabilities and in a few studies with individuals with severe disabilities (Kagohara 2011; Kagohara et al. 2011). They appear to be effective for tasks that do not have a large number of sequential steps. Palmtop-based job prompts were used in a series of studies with individuals who functioned in the severe range of intellectual disabilities (Furniss et al. 2001). Although successful, there have been no follow-up studies attesting to a wider use of this instructional prompt system. It has the advantage of being small, portable, and relatively inexpensive. The use of electronic control devices that produce visual, auditory, or mechanical (e.g., air blowing) prompts has been found to be rather effective in teaching individuals with very severe disabilities to engage in simple occupational and vocational tasks.

The use of assistive electronic technology is in its nascent stages as applied to instructional prompts for occupational and vocational training in this population. Thus, the field is open to further research. For example, Lancioni et al. (1999a) assessed whether instructions can be grouped following initial acquisition of a skill via palmtop-based instructions so that the number of instruction can be reduced. They found the individuals were able to maintain a high level of correct performance even under this condition. Similar efficiencies can be researched with other assistive technology instructional prompts (such as audio prompts). In addition, there has been a dearth of comparison studies across different instructional modalities in people with severe to profound intellectual disabilities to determine which procedures work best and under what conditions.

Another important research area is the assessment of attitudes of caregivers, family members, and the individuals toward different assistive technologies. For example, some caregivers may consider the use of self-verbalizations a preferable strategy because it does not require the individuals to depend on external cues and allows them to appear more in control of the situation and more autonomous (Hughes and Agran 1993), while others may find it to be a difficult and time consuming strategy and a relatively artificial approach with individuals who have limited receptive language (Storey and Provost 1996). Furthermore, the individuals may have specific preferences themselves that they may find more motivating to engage in than a lesser preferred instructional strategy (Lancioni et al. 1999b).

Leisure Skills

If given a choice, most individuals would undoubtedly choose to engage in leisure activities that give them pleasure and increase their happiness (Helm 2000). Individuals with severe/profound or multiple disabilities have limited choices in terms of leisure activities they can access that makes them happy (Green and Reid 1999; Lancioni et al. 2005c). Their choices are apparently inversely related to the degree of their cognitive and physical impairments; their disabilities restrict their response repertoire that, in turn, reduces their opportunities for constructive engagement with their environment. Thus, researchers have been very active in developing assistive technology options that can increase their choice of leisure activities (Lancioni et al. 2008a). These have included the identification and assessment of new responses and matching microswitches that might allow a person with minimal motor movement to benefit from microswitch programs and the availability of multiple microswitches to exercise choice (Lancioni et al. 2005b).

There has been a plethora of studies that have assessed the utility of single and multiple microswitches that allow individuals to access single or multiple leisure activities (see also Chap. 2). Results reported in these studies were generally very positive, indicating that individuals with a range of severe physical and intellectual disabilities could learn to use the microswitches and to make choices among alternative leisure activities. The unique aspect of this research is that it encompassed individuals with a vast array of minimal motor responses that could be used to develop movement-specific individualized microswitches, which enabled the person to access stimulation. Indeed, virtually every body part has been used to operate microswitches.

The majority of the microswitch studies demonstrated the utility of the microswitches to access brief stimulation. However, a minority of the studies included assistive technology to enable the individuals to actually engage in the leisure activities for longer durations of their choice. These studies used assistive technology to enable individuals to self-operate such devices as a radio, television, and iPod Touch® to listen to music or watch entertainment programs. In addition, a few studies explored the use of computers to write e-mail to family and friends, or use technology to send and receive electronic messaging, thereby expanding the individual's social horizon beyond the confines of the wheelchair or bed.

Using microswitches as a tool to access stimulation or leisure activities, or using assistive technology to operate devices for entertainment is an emerging field. In addition to finding easy-to-use and physical energy-efficient personalized microswitches, future research should assess new assistive technologies for enabling individuals with severe/profound and multiple disabilities to access and use electronic devices, including smart phones; HD television; portable media players (e.g., MP3 players and iPods) for music, video, and picture taking; and computer tablets (e.g., iPad) for a large range of leisure activities, including texting and social networking. The room for new research initiatives in this area appears to be boundless.

References

Agran, M., Fodor-Davis, J., & Moore, S. (1986). The effects of self-instructional training on job-task sequencing: Suggesting a problem-solving strategy. *Education and Training of the Mentally Retarded, 21*, 273–281.

Agran, M., Fodor-Davis, J., Moore, S., & Martella, R. C. (1992). Effects of peer-delivered self-instructional training on a lunch-making work task for students with severe disabilities. *Education and Training in Mental Retardation, 27*, 230–240.

Alberto, P. A., Sharpton, W. R., Briggs, A., & Stright, M. H. (1986). Facilitating task acquisition through the use of self-operated auditory prompting system. *Journal of the Association for Persons with Severe Handicaps, 11*, 85–91.

Alberto, P. A., Cihak, D. F., & Gama, R. I. (2005). Use of static picture prompts versus video modeling during simulation instruction. *Research in Developmental Disabilities, 26*, 327–339.

Algozzine, B., Browder, D., Karvonen, M., Test, D. W., & Wood, W. M. (2001). Effects of interventions to promote self-determination for individuals with disabilities. *Review of Educational Research, 71*, 219–277.

Anderson, M. D., Sherman, J. A., Sheldon, J. B., & McAdam, D. (1997). Picture activity schedules and engagement of adults with mental retardation in a group home. *Research in Developmental Disabilities, 18*, 231–250.

Anson, D., Moist, P., Przywara, M., Wells, H., Saylor, H., & Maxime, H. (2006). The effects of word completion and word prediction on typing rates using on-screen keyboards. *Assistive Technology, 18*, 146–154.

Antonucci, M., Lancioni, G. E., Singh, N. N., O'Reilly, M. F., Sigafoos, J., Oliva, D., & Bosco, A. (2006). A writing program with word prediction for a young adult with multiple disabilities: A preliminary assessment. *Perceptual and Motor Skills, 103*, 223–228.

Bache, J., & Derwent, G. (2008). Access to computer-based leisure for individuals with profound disabilities. *NeuroRehabilitation, 23*, 343–350.

Baker, P. M., & Moon, N. W. (2008). Wireless technologies and accessibility for people with disabilities: Findings from a policy research instrument. *Assistive Technology, 20*, 149–156.

Barlow, D. H., Nock, M., & Hersen, M. (2009). *Single-case experimental designs* (3rd ed.). New York: Allyn & Bacon.

Barnard, K., & Johnson, M. (2005). Word sense disambiguation with pictures. *Artificial Intelligence, 167*, 13–30.

Berg, W. K., & Wacker, D. P. (1989). Evaluation of tactile prompts with a student who is deaf, blind, and mentally retarded. *Journal of Applied Behavior Analysis, 22*, 93–99.

Betke, M., Gips, J., & Fleming, P. (2002). The camera mouse: Visual tracking of body features to provide computer access for people with severe disabilities. *IEEE Transactions on Rehabilitation Engineering, 10*, 1–10.

Briggs, A., Alberto, P., Sharpton, W., Berlin, K., McKinley, C., & Ritts, C. (1990). Generalized use of a self-operated audio prompt system. *Education and Training in Mental Retardation, 21*, 381–389.

Brodwin, M. G., Cardoso, E., & Star, T. (2004). Computer assistive technology for people who have disabilities: Computer adaptations and modifications. *Journal of Rehabilitation, 70*, 28–33.

Browder, D. M., & Shapiro, E. S. (1985). Application of self-management to individuals with severe handicaps: A review. *Journal of the Association for Persons with Severe Handicaps, 10*, 200–208.

Brown, L., Branston, M., Hamre-Nietupski, S., Pumpian, I., Certo, N., & Gruenewald, L. (1979). A strategy for developing chronological-age appropriate and functional curricular content for severely handicapped adolescents and young adults. *The Journal of Special Education, 13*, 81–90.

Callahan, K., Henson, R. K., & Cowan, A. K. (2008). Social validation of evidence-based practices in autism by parents, teachers, and administrators. *Journal of Autism and Developmental Disorders, 38*, 678–692.

Chen, Y. L. (2001). Application of tilt sensors in human-computer mouse interface for people with disabilities. *IEEE Transactions on Rehabilitation Engineering, 9*, 289–294.

Cihak, D., Alberto, P. A., Taber-Doughty, T., & Gama, R. I. (2006a). A comparison of static picture prompting and video prompting simulation strategies using group instructional procedures. *Focus on Autism and Other Developmental Disabilities, 21*, 89–99.

Cihak, D. F., Kessler, K. B., & Alberto, P. A. (2006b). Generalized use of a handheld prompting system. *Research in Developmental Disabilities, 28*, 397–408.

Connis, R. (1979). The effects of sequential pictorial cues, self-recording, and praise on the job task sequencing of retarded adults. *Journal of Applied Behavior Analysis, 12*, 355–361.

Crawford, M. R., & Schuster, J. W. (1993). Using microswitches to teach toy use. *Journal of Developmental and Physical Disabilities, 5*, 349–368.

Cuvo, A., Leaf, R., & Borakove, L. (1978). Teaching janitorial skills to the mentally retarded: Acquisition, generalization, and maintenance. *Journal of Applied Behavior Analysis, 11*, 345–355.

Dattilo, J., & Schleien, S. J. (1994). Understanding leisure services for individuals with mental retardation. *Mental Retardation, 32*, 53–59.

Davies, D. K., Stock, S., & Wehmeyer, M. L. (2002a). Enhancing independent task performance for individuals with mental retardation through the use of a handheld self-directed visual and audio programming system. *Education and Training in Mental Retardation and Developmental Disabilities, 37*, 209–218.

Davies, D. K., Stock, S., & Wehmeyer, M. L. (2002b). Enhancing independent time-management skills of individuals with mental retardation using a palmtop personal computer. *Mental Retardation, 40*, 358–365.

Davies, D. K., Stock, S., & Wehmeyer, M. L. (2003). A palmtop computer-based intelligent aid for individuals with intellectual disabilities to increase independent decision making. *Research and Practice for Persons with Severe Disabilities, 28*, 182–193.

Davis, C. A., Brady, M. P., Williams, R. E., & Burta, M. (1992). The effects of self-operated auditory prompting tapes on the performance fluency of persons with severe mental retardation. *Education and Training in Mental Retardation, 22*, 39–50.

Dixon, L. S. (1981). A functional analysis of photo-object matching skills of severely retarded adolescents. *Journal of Applied Behavior Analysis, 14*, 465–478.

Edrisinha, C., O'Reilly, M. F., Choi, H. Y., Sigafoos, J., & Lancioni, G. E. (2011). "Say Cheese": Teaching photography skills to adults with developmental disabilities. *Research in Developmental Disabilities, 32*, 636–642.

Egan, J. M., Chenoweth, L., & McAuliffe, D. (2006). E-mail-facilitated qualitative interviews with traumatic brain injury survivors: A new and accessible method. *Brain Injury, 20*, 1283–1294.

Evans, D. G., Drew, R., & Blenkhorn, P. (2000). Controlling mouse pointer position using an infrared head-operated joystick. *IEEE Transactions on Rehabilitation Engineering, 8*, 107–117.

Furniss, F., Ward, A., Lancioni, G., Rocha, N., Cunha, B., Seedhouse, P., Morato, P., & Waddell, N. (1999). A palmtop-based job aid for workers with severe intellectual disabilities. *Technology and Disability, 10*, 53–67.

Furniss, F., Lancioni, G. E., Rocha, N., Cunha, B., Seedhouse, P., Morato, P., & O'Reilly, M. F. (2001). VICAID: Development and evaluation of a palm-top job aid for workers with severe developmental disabilities. *British Journal of Educational Technology, 32*, 277–287.

Gartland, D. (2004). Considerations in the selection and use of technology with people who have cognitive deficits following acquired brain injury. *Neuropsychological Rehabilitation, 14*, 61–75.

Goodson, J., Sigafoos, J., O'Reilly, M., Canella, H., & Lancioni, G. E. (2007). Evaluation of a video-based error correction procedure for teaching a domestic skill to individuals with developmental disabilities. *Research in Developmental Disabilities, 28*, 458–467.

Green, C. W., & Reid, D. H. (1999). A behavioral approach to identifying sources of happiness and unhappiness among individuals with profound disabilities. *Behavior Modification, 23*, 280–293.

Helm, D. T. (2000). The measurement of happiness. *American Journal on Mental Retardation, 105*, 326–335.

Horner, R., & McDonald, R. (1982). Comparison of single instance and general case instruction in teaching a generalized vocational skill. *The Journal of the Association for the Severely Handicapped, 7*, 7–20.

Hughes, C., & Agran, M. (1993). Teaching persons with severe disabilities to use self-instruction in community settings: An analysis of applications. *Journal of the Association for Persons with Severe Handicaps, 18*, 261–274.

Hunter, J., & Bellamy, G. (1976). Cable harness construction for severely retarded adults: A demonstration of training techniques. *American Association for the Education of Severely/Profoundly Handicapped Review, 1*, 2–13.

Joseph, L. M., & Konrad, M. (2009). Teaching students with intellectual or developmental disabilities to write: A review of the literature. *Research in Developmental Disabilities, 30*, 1–19.

Kagohara, D. M. (2011). Three students with developmental disabilities learn to operate an iPod to access age-appropriate entertainment videos. *Journal of Behavioral Education, 20*, 33–43.

Kagohara, D. M., Sigafoos, J., Achmadi, D., van der Meer, L., O'Reilly, M. F., & Lancioni, G. E. (2011). Teaching students with developmental disabilities to operate an iPod Touch® to listen to music. *Research in Developmental Disabilities, 32*, 2987–2992.

Lancioni, G. E., & O'Reilly, M. F. (2001). Self-management of instruction cues for occupation: Review of studies with people with severe and profound disabilities. *Research in Developmental Disabilities, 22*, 41–65.

Lancioni, G. E., & Oliva, D. (1988). A computer-aided programme for promoting unsupervised activities for multihandicapped adolescents. *Journal of Mental Deficiency Research, 32*, 125–136.

Lancioni, G. E., Van den Hof, E., Boelens, H., Rocha, N., & Seedhouse, P. (1998). A computer-based system providing pictorial instructions and prompts to promote task performance in persons with severe developmental disabilities. *Behavioral Interventions, 13*, 111–122.

Lancioni, G. E., O'Reilly, M. F., Van den Hof, E., Furniss, F., Seedhouse, P., & Rocha, N. (1999a). Task instructions for persons with severe intellectual disability: Reducing the number of occasions after the acquisition. *Behavioral Interventions, 14*, 199–211.

Lancioni, G. E., Van den Hof, E., Furniss, F., O'Reilly, M. F., & Cunha, B. (1999b). Evaluation of a computer-aided system providing pictorial task instructions and prompts to people with severe intellectual disability. *Journal of Intellectual Disability Research, 43*, 61–66.

Lancioni, G. E., O'Reilly, M. F., Seedhouse, P., Furniss, F., & Cunha, B. (2000). Promoting independent task performance by persons with severe developmental disabilities through a new computer-aided system. *Behavior Modification, 24*, 700–718.

Lancioni, G. E., O'Reilly, M. F., & Oliva, D. (2001). Instruction strategies for promoting vocational activities: A preliminary assessment of preferences with persons with multiple disabilities. *Journal of Developmental and Physical Disabilities, 9*, 79–89.

Lancioni, G. E., Singh, N. N., O'Reilly, M. F., Oliva, D., Montironi, G., Piazza, F., Ciavattini, E., & Bettarelli, F. (2004). Using computer systems as microswitches for vocal utterances of persons with multiple disabilities. *Research in Developmental Disabilities, 25*, 183–192.

Lancioni, G. E., Singh, N. N., O'Reilly, M. F., & Oliva, D. (2005a). Microswitch programs for persons with multiple disabilities: An overview of the responses adopted for microswitch activation. *Cognitive Processing, 6*, 177–188.

Lancioni, G. E., Singh, N. N., O'Reilly, M. F., & Oliva, D. (2005b). Using a hand-tap response with a vibration microswitch with students with multiple disabilities. *Behavioural and Cognitive Psychotherapy, 30*, 237–241.

Lancioni, G. E., Singh, N. N., O'Reilly, M. F., Oliva, D., & Basili, G. (2005c). An overview of research on increasing indices of happiness of people with severe/profound intellectual and multiple disabilities. *Disability and Rehabilitation, 27*, 83–93.

Lancioni, G. E., Singh, N. N., O'Reilly, M. F., Sigafoos, J., Oliva, D., Costantini, A., Gatto, S., Marinelli, V., & Putzolu, A. (2006). An optic microswitch for an eyelid response to foster environmental control in children with minimal motor behavior. *Pediatric Rehabilitation, 9*, 53–56.

Lancioni, G. E., O'Reilly, M. F., Singh, N. N., Sigafoos, J., Chiapparino, C., Stasolla, F., Bosco, A., De Pace, C., & Oliva, D. (2007a). Enabling a young man with minimal motor behavior to manage independently his leisure television engagement. *Perceptual and Motor Skills, 104*, 47–54.

Lancioni, G. E., Singh, N. N., O'Reilly, M. F., Sigafoos, J., Chiapparino, C., Stasolla, F., & Oliva, D. (2007b). Using an optic sensor and a scanning keyboard emulator to facilitate writing by persons with pervasive motor disabilities. *Journal of Developmental and Physical Disabilities, 19*, 593–603.

Lancioni, G. E., Tota, A., Smaldone, A., Singh, N. N., O'Reilly, M. F., Sigafoos, J., Oliva, D., & Montironi, G. (2007c). Extending the evaluation of novel microswitch technology for small responses in children with profound multiple disabilities. *Assistive Technology, 19*, 11–16.

Lancioni, G. E., O'Reilly, M. F., Singh, N. N., Sigafoos, J., Oliva, D., Antonucci, M., Tota, A., & Basili, G. (2008a). Microswitch-based programs for persons with multiple disabilities: An overview of some recent developments. *Perceptual and Motor Skills, 106*, 355–370.

Lancioni, G. E., Singh, N. N., O'Reilly, M. F., Sigafoos, J., Oliva, D., Campodonico, F., & Groeneweg, J. (2008b). Assisting persons with multiple disabilities to move through simple occupational activities with automatic prompting. *Research in Developmental Disabilities, 29*, 439–446.

Lancioni, G. E., Singh, N. N., O'Reilly, M. F., Sigafoos, J., Green, V., Chiapparino, C., Stasolla, F., & Oliva, D. (2009). A voice-detecting sensor and a scanning keyboard emulator to support word writing by two boys with extensive motor disabilities. *Research in Developmental Disabilities, 30*, 203–209.

Lancioni, G. E., O'Reilly, M. F., Singh, N. N., Green, V., Chiapparino, C., De Pace, C., Alberti, G., & Stasolla, F. (2010a). Use of microswitch technology and a keyboard emulator to support literacy performance of persons with extensive neuro-motor disabilities. *Developmental Neurorehabilitation, 13*, 248–257.

Lancioni, G. E., Singh, N. N., O'Reilly, M. F., Sigafoos, J., Oliva, D., Signorino, M., & De Tommaso, M. (2010b). Helping a man with acquired brain injury and multiple disabilities manage television use via assistive technology. *Clinical Case Studies, 9*, 285–293.

Lancioni, G. E., Singh, N. N., O'Reilly, M. F., Sigafoos, J., Signorino, S., Oliva, D., Alberti, G., Carrella, L., & De Tommaso, M. (2010c). A special messaging technology for two persons with acquired brain injury and multiple disabilities. *Brain Injury, 24*, 1236–1243.

Lancioni, G. E., Singh, N. N., O'Reilly, M. F., Zonno, N., Cassano, G., De Vanna, F., De Bari, A. L., Pinto, K., & Minervini, M. (2010d). Persons with Alzheimer's disease perform daily activities using verbal-instruction technology: A maintenance assessment. *Developmental Neurorehabilitation, 13*, 103–113.

Lancioni, G. E., Bellini, D., Oliva, D., Singh, N. N., O'Reilly, M. F., Lang, R., & Didden, R. (2011a). Camera-based microswitch technology to monitor mouth, eyebrow, and eyelid responses of children with profound multiple disabilities. *Journal of Behavioral Education, 20*, 4–14.

Lancioni, G. E., O'Reilly, M. F., Singh, N. N., Buonocunto, F., Sacco, V., Colonna, F., Navarro, J., Oliva, D., & Megna, M. (2011b). Technology-assisted opportunities for two persons emerged from a minimally conscious state and showing extensive motor disabilities. *Developmental Neurorehabilitation, 14*, 8–14.

Lancioni, G. E., O'Reilly, M. F., Singh, N. N., Oliva, D., Buonocunto, F., & Belardinelli, M. O. (2011c). Technology-assisted writing opportunities for a man emerged from a minimally conscious state and affected by extensive motor disabilities. *Developmental Neurorehabilitation, 14*, 123–127.

Lancioni, G. E., O'Reilly, M. F., Singh, N. N., Sigafoos, J., Oliva, D., Buonocunto, F., & Belardinelli, M. O. (2011d). Technology assisted writing opportunities for a man emerged from a minimally conscious state and affected by extensive motor disabilities. *Developmental Neurorehabilitation, 14*, 123–127.

Lancioni, G. E., O'Reilly, M. F., Singh, N. N., Sigafoos, J., Oliva, D., Smaldone, A., La Martire, M. L., Navarro, J., Spica, A., & Chirico, M. (2011e). Technology-assisted programs for promoting leisure or communication engagement in two persons with pervasive motor or multiple disabilities. *Disability and Rehabilitation: Assistive Technology, 6*, 108–114.

Lancioni, G. E., Singh, N. N., O'Reilly, M. F., & Sigafoos, J. (2011f). Assistive technology for behavioral interventions for persons with severe/profound multiple disabilities: A selective overview. *European Journal of Behavior Analysis, 12*, 7–26.

Lancioni, G. E., Singh, N. N., O'Reilly, M. F., Sigafoos, J., Green, V., Oliva, D., & Lang, R. (2011g). Microswitch and keyboard-emulator technology to facilitate the writing performance of persons with extensive motor disabilities. *Research in Developmental Disabilities, 32*, 576–582.

Lancioni, G. E., Singh, N. N., O'Reilly, M. F., Sigafoos, J., & Oliva, D. (2011h). A verbal-instruction system to help a woman with intellectual disability and blindness manage food- and drink-preparation tasks. *Clinical Case Studies, 10*, 79–90.

Lancioni, G. E., Singh, N. N., O'Reilly, M. F., Sigafoos, J., Oliva, D., Smaldone, A., La Martire, M. L., Alberti, G., & Scigliuzzo, F. (2011i). A verbal-instruction system to help persons with multiple disabilities to perform complex food- and drink-preparation tasks independently. *Research in Developmental Disabilities, 32*, 2739–2747.

Lasater, M. W., & Brady, M. P. (1995). Effects of video self-modeling and feedback on task fluency: A home-based intervention. *Education and Treatment of Children, 18*, 389–408.

LeGrice, B., & Blampied, N. M. (1994). Training pupils with intellectual disabilities educational technology using video prompting. *Education and Training in Mental Retardation and Developmental Disabilities, 29*, 321–330.

Martin, J. E., Mithaug, D. E., & Frazier, E. S. (1992). Effects of picture references on PVC chair, love seat, and settee assemblies by students with mental retardation. *Research in Developmental Disabilities, 13*, 267–286.

McLean, L. K., Brady, N. C., McLean, J. E., & Behrens, G. A. (1999). Communication forms and functions of children and adults with severe mental retardation in community and institutional settings. *Journal of Speech, Language, and Hearing Research, 42*, 231–240.

Mechling, L. C. (2006). Comparison of the effects of three approaches on the frequency of stimulus activation, via a single switch, by students with profound intellectual disabilities. *The Journal of Special Education, 40*, 94–102.

Moisey, S., & van de Keere, R. (2007). Inclusion and the Internet: Teaching adults with developmental disabilities to use information and communication technology. *Developmental Disabilities Bulletin, 35*, 72–102.

Moore, S. C., Agran, M., & Fodor-Davis, J. (1989). Using self-management strategies to increase the production rates of workers with severe handicaps. *Education and Training in Mental Retardation, 24*, 324–333.

Riffel, L. A., Wehmeyer, M. L., Turnbull, A. P., Lattimore, J., Davies, D., Stock, S., & Fisher, S. (2005). Promoting independent performance of transition-related tasks using a palmtop pc-based self-directed visual and auditory prompting system. *Journal of Special Education Technology, 20*, 5–14.

Rusch, F. R. (1986). Developing a long-term follow-up program. In F. R. Rusch (Ed.), *Competitive employment issues and strategies* (pp. 225–232). Baltimore: Paul H. Brookes.

Salend, S. J., Ellis, L. L., & Reynolds, C. J. (1989). Using self-instruction to teach vocational skills to individuals who are severely retarded. *Education and Training in Mental Retardation, 24*, 248–254.

Schleien, S. J., Meyer, S., Heyne, L., & Brandt, B. (1995). *Lifelong leisure skills and lifestyles for persons with developmental disabilities*. Baltimore: Brookes.

Simpson, T., Gauthier, M., & Prochazka, A. (2010). Evaluation of tooth-click triggering and speech recognition in assistive technology for computer access. *Neurorehabilitation and Neural Repair, 24*, 188–194.

Singh, N. N., Oswald, D. P., Ellis, C. R., & Singh, S. D. (1995). Community-based instruction for independent meal preparation by adults with profound mental retardation. *Journal of Behavioral Education, 5*, 77–91.

Sowers, J., Rusch, F., Connis, R., & Cummings, L. (1980). Teaching mentally retarded adults to time manage in a vocational setting. *Journal of Applied Behavior Analysis, 13*, 119–128.

Sowers, J., Verdi, M., Bourbeau, P., & Sheehan, M. (1985). Teaching job independence and flexibility to mentally retarded students through the use of self-control package. *Journal of Applied Behavior Analysis, 18*, 81–85.

Steed, S. E., & Lutzker, J. R. (1999). Recorded audio prompts: A strategy to increase independent prevocational task completion in individuals with dual diagnosis. *Behavior Modification, 23*, 152–168.

Storey, K., & Provost, O. (1996). The effect of communication skills instruction on the integration of workers with severe disabilities in supported employment settings. *Education and Training in Mental Retardation and Developmental Disabilities, 31*, 123–141.

Tam, C., Reid, D., Naumann, S., & O'Keefe, B. (2002). Perceived benefits of word prediction intervention on written productivity in children with spina bifida and hydrocephalus. *Occupational Therapy International, 9*, 237–255.

Taylor, R. G. (1987). Teaching a severely handicapped deaf-blind young woman to prepare breakfast foods. *Journal of Visual Impairment and Blindness, 81*, 67–69.

Todis, B., Sohlberg, M. M., Hood, D., & Fickas, S. (2005). Making electronic mail accessible: Perspectives of people with acquired cognitive impairments, caregivers and professionals. *Brain Injury, 19*, 389–401.

Tota, A., Lancioni, G. E., Singh, N. N., O'Reilly, M. F., Sigafoos, J., & Oliva, D. (2006). Evaluating the applicability of optic microswitches for eyelid responses in students with profound multiple disabilities. *Disability and Rehabilitation: Assistive Technology, 1*, 217–223.

Turpin, G., Armstrong, J., Frost, P., Fine, B., Wards, C. D., & Pinnington, L. L. (2005). Evaluation of alternative computer input devices used by people with disabilities. *Journal of Medical Engineering & Technology, 29*, 119–129.

Varona, J., Manrea-Yee, C., & Perales, F. J. (2008). Hands-free vision-based interface for computer accessibility. *Journal of Network and Computer Application, 31*, 357–374.

Wacker, D. P., & Berg, W. (1983). Effects of picture prompts on the acquisition of complex vocational tasks independently by mentally retarded adolescents. *Journal of Applied Behavior Analysis, 16*, 417–433.

Wacker, D. P., & Berg, W. K. (1984). Training adolescents with severe handicaps to set up job tasks independently using picture prompts. *Analysis and Intervention in Developmental Disabilities, 4*, 353–365.

Wacker, D. P., Berg, W. K., Berrie, P., & Swatta, P. (1985). Generalization and maintenance of complex skills by severely handicapped adolescents following picture prompt training. *Journal of Applied Behavior Analysis, 18*, 329–336.

Wehmeyer, M. L., & Field, S. (2007). *Self-determination: Instructional and assessment strategies*. Thousand Oaks: Corwin Press.

Wehmeyer, M. L., Palmer, S. B., Smith, S. J., Parent, W., Davies, D. K., & Stock, S. (2006). Technology use by people with intellectual and developmental disabilities to support employment activities: A single-subject design meta analysis. *Journal of Vocational Rehabilitation, 24*, 81–86.

Wehmeyer, M. L., Agran, M., Hughes, C., Martin, J., Mithaug, D. E., & Palmer, S. (2007). *Promoting self-determination in students with intellectual and developmental disabilities*. New York: Guilford Press.

Williams, S. C. (2002). How speech feedback and word prediction software can help students write. *Teaching Exceptional Children, 34*, 72–78.

Wilson, P. G., Schepis, M. M., & Mason-Main, M. (1987). In vivo use of picture prompt training to increase independent work at a restaurant. *The Journal of the Association for Persons with Severe Handicaps, 12*, 145–150.

Chapter 5
Orientation Systems for Promoting Indoor Travel

Abstract This chapter provides an overview of studies assessing the use of orientation systems to help persons with severe/profound and multiple disabilities (including persons with Alzheimer's disease) travel to indoor destinations independently. The first part of this chapter analyzes the studies that used orientation systems relying on direction cues. The studies were divided based on the types of cues employed, that is, auditory (buzzer-like) sounds, verbal messages (without and with procedural extensions), and visual cues. The second part of this chapter analyzes the few studies that used orientation systems relying on corrective feedback. The final part of this chapter analyzes the outcomes of the studies reviewed and their implications for daily programs, examines practical aspects concerning the use of the systems, and suggests questions for new research in the area.

Introduction

Orientation and mobility problems within indoor daily contexts are common among (a) persons with severe visual impairment and other disabilities, such as neuromotor and intellectual disabilities, as well as (b) persons without severe visual impairment but with profound intellectual disabilities or degenerative neurological syndromes (e.g., Alzheimer's disease) (Gadler et al. 2009; Joffee and Rikhye 1991; Lancioni et al. 1995a, b, 1996b, 2000b, 2010a, b, 2011; Marquardt and Schmieg 2009; Provencher et al. 2008; Uslan et al. 1983, 1988). These problems can have serious negative implications for the persons affected, namely, they can interfere with and reduce the persons' activity engagement, curtail their independence, limit (damage) their self-assurance, and ultimately depress their developmental and social opportunities and general mood (Algozzine et al. 2001; Karvonen et al. 2004; Konrad et al. 2007; Lachapelle et al. 2005; Lancioni et al. 2000a, b; Petry et al. 2005, 2009; Provencher et al. 2008).

G.E. Lancioni et al., *Assistive Technology: Interventions for Individuals with Severe/Profound and Multiple Disabilities*, Autism and Child Psychopathology Series, DOI 10.1007/978-1-4614-4229-5_5, © Springer Science+Business Media New York 2013

In light of the negative implications of orientation and travel problems, there is wide consensus on the general need to address such problems and improve the situation of the persons affected by them (Draheim et al. 2002; Gibson et al. 2004; Higgerty and Williams 2005; Lancioni et al. 2007; Rainville et al. 2001). The strategies suggested to this end vary substantially, and their suitability for persons with severe/profound and multiple disabilities and their caregivers may also be largely different. For example, teaching the persons to use tactile maps, that is, miniature replicas of the travel area and possible landmarks characterizing it (as orientation material), may prove too difficult for persons with profound intellectual disabilities. These persons would easily fail to discriminate the distinctive/characteristic features of the replicas or to relate them to the corresponding features of the real context (Cherrier et al. 2001; Joffee 1995; Lancioni et al. 2007; Martinsen et al. 2007). Similar problems could also be found with persons with direction and laterality problems (Guth and LaDuke 1994, 1995; Lancioni et al. 2007). The use of auditory maps, that is, verbal descriptions of the environment as illustration and guidance cues, would not resolve the problems mentioned above. To the contrary, it could add extra difficulties, as many of these persons would not be able to discriminate and utilize verbal cues (Lancioni et al. 2008).

The use of backward-chaining strategies to teach specific routes may have some potential as well as some clear limits (Kazdin 2001). Those strategies begin by promoting independence on the last portion of a route to a specific (relevant) destination. Once the person achieves independence on this portion, the intervention focuses on gradually extending the length of space that he or she can manage independently (i.e., adds a new portion to the last of the route that the person already possessed) (Jerome et al. 2007; Lancioni et al. 2011; McGilton et al. 2003; Provencher et al. 2008). Eventually, the intervention would target the entire route. The main problems with these strategies are (a) the high implementation cost (i.e., the relatively long time required to teach the travel skill), (b) the frequent lack of generalization (i.e., the effects of teaching are generally specific/limited to the route on which it was applied and fail to generalize to other routes), and (c) a declining effectiveness of the intervention as the number of routes in the program increases (i.e., due to discrimination difficulties and confusion risks) (Brooks et al. 1999; Lancioni et al. 2011; Martelli et al. 2008).

A possible alternative to the aforementioned approaches may be represented by the use of assistive orientation technology (Baldwin 2003; Lancioni et al. 2007; Parker 2009; Ross and Kelly 2009). Early research on an assistive technology system, which was to promote orientation in persons with profound intellectual and multiple disabilities, was conducted by Uslan and his associates (Uslan 1976; Uslan et al. 1983, 1988). Their system was designed to provide auditory (musical) stimuli as spatial cues for orientation and travel. It included (a) a central electronic unit allowing the selection of the destinations to reach, (b) electronic floor sensors that were triggered by the participants while walking on them (and as a result activated auditory/musical cues), and a number of loudspeakers, which were along the routes to the destinations and served to emit the cues. The results were reported to be positive in terms of the system's effectiveness to guide the participants to the destinations. Nevertheless, some reservations were expressed as to the general practicality of the system, as it required that staff and participants always return to the starting point (i.e., to the central electronic unit) to select a new destination.

This early research was the basis for a variety of new studies aimed at building/improving on the technology and results presented by Uslan and associates. Some of the new studies focused on the development of a mobile robot to guide/support the participant to different destinations (i.e., according to the selection made by staff or by the participant on his or her own at each new travel instance) (Lancioni et al. 1993a, b, 1994b). The selection was made on the robot (through modified keys that could be discriminated and used also by persons with blindness and severe/profound intellectual disabilities). The robot seemed quite effective in terms of guidance and support for the participants but also presented serious drawbacks. For example, it was quite expensive, not easily transportable from one place to another, and not suitable for environments with drop-offs or stairs (Lancioni et al. 1995a, b, 2007).

Other studies (in addition to those focused on the development of the robot) were directed at assessing various orientation technology solutions that could respond to different personal needs (Lancioni et al. 1995a, b, 2008, 2009b). The basic reasoning was that persons who are blind and have a very limited notion of space and virtually no orientation abilities might benefit most from a system that does not require much initiative and self-direction from them (Lancioni et al. 2007). Such a system could be envisaged as one that provides direction cues, that is, cues that guide the person's travel by marking/specifying the space to the destination (Lancioni et al. 2007, 2010b). On the contrary, persons who have functional vision and/or possess a general notion of the spatial reality surrounding them could resort to a system that is less intrusive than the one mentioned above. This latter system would not resort to directive cues but would simply employ corrective feedback. Specifically, the person would be allowed to engage in travel using his or her self-management and initiative skills (Lancioni et al. 2009b). The system would only intervene in case the person deviates from or loses the correct direction. In that case, a feedback would be presented that lasts until the person has found the correct direction again.

This chapter provides an overview of studies assessing orientation systems to help persons with severe/profound and multiple disabilities (including persons with Alzheimer's disease) travel to indoor destinations independently. The first part of this chapter analyzes the studies that used assistive orientation technology involving direction cues. The studies were divided based on the types of cues employed, that is, auditory (buzzer-like) sounds, verbal messages (without and with procedural extensions), and visual cues. The second part of this chapter analyzes the few studies that used assistive orientation technology involving corrective feedback. The final part of this chapter analyzes (discusses) the outcomes of the studies reviewed and their implications for daily programs, examines practical aspects concerning

Table 5.1 Studies of orientation systems with direction cues grouped according to the types of cues used

Studies	Participants	Age (years)	Cues used
Lancioni et al. (1995a)	4	12.5–15	Auditory (buzzer-like) cues
Lancioni et al. (1996a)	2	17, 28	Auditory (buzzer-like) cues
Lancioni et al. (1998b)	2	16, 17	Auditory (buzzer-like) cues
Lancioni et al. (1997b)	2	17, 19	Auditory (verbal-message) cues
Lancioni et al. (1998d)	1	19	Auditory (verbal-message) cues
Lancioni et al. (1999a)	2	30, 32	Auditory (verbal-message) cues
Lancioni et al. (2001)	2	18, 21	Auditory (verbal-message) cues
Lancioni et al. (2008)	2	28, 38	Auditory (verbal-message) cues
Lancioni et al. (2010a)	4	32–50	Auditory (verbal-message) cues
Lancioni et al. (2010b)	2	21, 24	Auditory (verbal-message) cues
Lancioni et al. (2011)	3	73–83	Auditory (verbal-message) cues
Lancioni and Mantini (1998)	2	31, 39	Auditory (verbal-message) cues with extensions
Lancioni et al. (2009a)	1	27	Auditory (verbal-message) cues with extensions
Lancioni and Oliva (1999)	1	18	Visual (light) cues
Lancioni et al. (1996c)	2	18, 19	Visual (light) cues
Lancioni et al. (1998a)	2	19, 27	Visual (light) cues
Lancioni et al. (1998c)	1	28	Visual (light) cues
Lancioni et al. (2000b)	1	35	Visual (light) cues

the use of the orientation technology systems reported, and suggests questions for new research in the area.

Studies of Orientation Systems with Direction Cues

Orientation systems relying on direction cues require the persons to follow in the direction of the cues and walk toward them (Lancioni et al. 2007). Generally, the cues are auditory signals and can consist of complex sound (buzzer-like) cues or verbal messages. A number of studies have also assessed the use of visual cues (lights). The cues are not continuous but repeated at intervals of different lengths to avoid habituation effects and reduce the level of disturbance in the context in which they occur (i.e., for the family/staff members or other patients available in that context). Table 5.1 presents a list of 18 studies grouped according to the type of cues they employed. The first three studies listed in the table involved the use of *auditory (buzzer-like) cues* (Lancioni et al. 1995a, 1996a, 1998b). The following eight studies of the table involved the use of *auditory (verbal-message) cues* (Lancioni et al. 1997b, 1998d, 1999a, 2001, 2008, 2010a, b, 2011). The next two studies involved the use of *auditory (verbal-message) cues* but with procedural extensions (Lancioni and Mantini 1998; Lancioni et al. 2009a). The last five studies involved the use of *visual (light) cues* (Lancioni and Oliva 1999; Lancioni et al. 1996c, 1998a, c, 2000b).

Auditory (Buzzer-Like) Cues

The study by Lancioni et al. (1995a) included four participants between 12.5 and 15 years of age who were totally blind and were considered to be functioning within the profound intellectual disability range. The participants were expected to travel to several indoor destinations for their daily activities, but their orientation was poor, and they required fairly consistent assistance from caregivers/staff. The technology involved a portable electronic control device and a variety of acoustic sources, which were used to mark the routes to the different destinations. Each acoustic source involved a coded radio receiver activated by a signal of the portable device, an electromagnetic generator for the proximity sensor of the portable device, and a battery. The portable device (worn by the participant at his chest) included selection keys, a coded radio transmitter, a proximity sensor, and a battery. Before each travel, the supervising staff person selected the route that the participant was to follow on the portable device. This was done by entering the route's identification number through the aforementioned selection keys. This operation could be carried out from any area where the participant was (rather than from a central selection unit, as it was the case in the studies by Uslan et al. 1983, 1988). Once the route had been entered, the first acoustic source available on that route (the closest to the participant's position) was activated. That is, it started emitting a complex harmonic sound with a perceived pitch of about 360 Hz, which alternated "on" and "off" phases of 3–5 s. When the participant came close to the source, the proximity sensor of the portable device deactivated that source and activated the next one in the route. The process was repeated until the last source (i.e., the one at the destination) was reached. Several sources could be used for the routes. Results showed that during baseline phases, the participants' percentages of correct travel were between 0 and about 30. During the last portion of the intervention, their percentages were near or above 90.

Lancioni et al. (1998b) carried out a study with two adolescents between 16 and 17 years of age who were diagnosed with total blindness and profound intellectual disabilities. The main goal of this study was to find a solution whereby the participants could be independent in entering the destinations that they were to reach into the portable device. Given that they would not be able to use the keys and digit the number codes (see above), the following conditions were arranged. First, the research assistant programmed a sequence of destinations within the portable device (i.e., memorized a series of number codes). Second, the device was provided with a front panel that worked as a switch. Third, at the start of the session and at each activity, the participant found a Velcro tag (a token to exchange for favorite items at the end of the session) that he was to attach to the front panel of the device. Pressing (attaching) this tag to the panel-switch activated the first acoustic source of the first/

next route programmed in the device. The participant was to reach that source and proceed as described above until he reached the destination. Both participants were successful in using the aforementioned Velcro tag solution. This ensured that they could be independent throughout the activity sessions (i.e., in entering the destinations and reaching them and in carrying out the activities scheduled at the destinations).

Auditory (Verbal-Message) Cues

In an attempt to make auditory cues less artificial, Lancioni et al. (1997b) replaced the buzzer-like sounds with spoken messages, which consisted of two to four words (e.g., the name of the participant and a word of encouragement). The message at the destinations also included words of praise. The messages were recorded by a person familiar to the participants and were emitted by the sound sources marking the routes (see above). The messages would occur at intervals of nearly 10 s until the participant had reached the destination. The system included the features to promote independence, described in relation to the article by Lancioni et al. (1998b). That is, the portable control system was programmed for a sequence of routes/destinations prior to the sessions, and its front panel was adapted as a switch for activating any of these routes/destinations according to the sequence preset. Moreover, the participants would find together with the object signals (i.e., the objects indicating the activity that they were to perform at the destinations) a Velcro tag serving as token to be attached to the front panel-switch of the device. The study, which was carried out with two boys of 17 and 19 years, showed that both participants learned to use the system and attend to the spoken cues very effectively and reached a percentage of correct travels exceeding 90. Their performance with the spoken cues matched the performance they displayed during comparison sessions in which the spoken messages were replaced with buzzer-like cues.

Lancioni et al. (1999a) carried out two case studies aimed at assessing a new version of the system designed for persons with limited attention and poor manipulation skills who could have difficulties finding the Velcro tag and attaching it to the front-switch part of the portable device. Such device allowed the staff/supervisor to program (a) the sequence of destinations (as described above) as well as (b) the intervals between the participant's arrival at a destination and the activation of the first source toward the next destination scheduled in the sequence. Activation of a source led to the emission of encouragement messages at intervals of nearly 10 s. When the participant reached a destination, the source there emitted a praise message and a timer in the portable device switched on. At the end of a preset interval (i.e., a time estimated to be sufficient for the participant to carry out the activity available at that destination), the device automatically activated the first source to the next destination. The participant was to follow the usual procedure by walking to that source and then continuing until he or she arrived at the next destination. Here, all the conditions described above were repeated (i.e., praise message, resetting of the timer, and eventually activation of the first source to the next destination). The two participants included in the case studies were a 30-year-old woman and a 32-year-old man. The first participant was highly successful with the program and reached levels of correct travels close to 100 %. The second participant also showed great improvement in performance. His mean level of correct travels exceeded 85 %.

Lancioni et al. (2010b) assessed an innovative portable device within an orientation program for two women of 24 and 21 years of age, respectively. The women were totally blind and presented with levels of intellectual disabilities estimated to be within the moderate or moderate to severe ranges. During each session, the women were to travel to six different destinations at each of which they were to carry out a familiar activity. The system involved the presence of a sound source at each of the destinations and a new portable device. This was a boxlike instrument of 20 cm × 15 cm × 4 cm that the participants had at their chest. The main (external) face of the box included six key areas, which corresponded to destinations to reach (activities to perform). Each of the key areas consisted of an embedded optic sensor covered with a discriminated (familiar) object representing the activity available at one of the destinations. As soon as the participant removed/detached an object for an activity (i.e., uncovering the underlying optic sensor), the sound source at the corresponding activity destination was activated. That is, brief encouragement messages were emitted at intervals of about 15 s until the participant reached the destination. At that point, the participant could receive verbal praise. The order with which the participants detached the objects from the portable device (selected the activities to carry out) depended totally on the participant's free will and self-determination. Both participants learned to use the system (and in particular the new portable device) rapidly and were successful in reaching the destinations and carrying out the activities available there. The participants also increased the speed with which they walked to the destinations over the course of the study.

Lancioni et al. (2011) reported the application of a basic version of the orientation program with three participants with Alzheimer's disease. The participants were between 73 and 83 years of age and had lost their abilities to carry out daily activities. Two of them were also diagnosed with mild levels of depression. All three participants attended a day center in which they were provided with some form of support for activity engagement. They had difficulties walking to different rooms of the center to engage in small activities or meet people and often required to be accompanied. The basic version of the program consisted in the supervisor activating the target destinations (one at a time) in the portable device and in the use of only one sound source per destination. The source emitted verbal (encouragement) messages at intervals of about 15 s. Two of the participants seemed able to orient to the messages/cues emitted by the sound sources and thus were introduced into the program directly. One did not seem capable of orienting to those messages/cues and was exposed to a preliminary intervention phase. At the beginning of this phase, the cues were presented at intervals of 5–6 s and were accompanied by the voice of the supervisor calling the person by name from the destination that was to be reached. When the person started to reach the destinations successfully under this condition, the interval between cues (and supervisor's calls) increased to about 10 s. Subsequently, the intervals were extended to 15 s, and the supervisor's voice was faded out. Data showed that the first two participants learned to use the system's cues very rapidly reaching a nearly errorless travel performance. The third participant benefited from the preliminary intervention phase and subsequently displayed a highly accurate travel performance similar to that of the first two participants.

Auditory (Verbal-Message) Cues with Program Extensions

The study by Lancioni and Mantini (1998) was aimed at evaluating an activity condition in which the orientation system was not used for a single person as in the other studies but for two persons simultaneously. The two persons were women of 39 and 31 years of age who had a diagnosis of total blindness, were rated in the profound intellectual disability range, and were familiar with the use of auditory orientation cues for indoor travel. The program was carried out in a multiroom setting, and sound sources with verbal messages were available to reach the destinations. One of the women wore the portable device in which the sequence of destinations to reach within the activity session was already programmed. The other woman wore a small box containing a radio and a proximity sensor. When the women approached a sound source on the way to a destination, the proximity sensor of either one of them was sufficient to deactivate that source and activate the next one. The source at the destination, however, continued to be active until it was approached by both women (i.e., until it was triggered by both proximity sensors). At the destination, each woman had an activity to carry out (i.e., one beside the other). Below the material for the activity, the women found an object signal indicating the next activity to carry out. The woman wearing the portable device was also to attach the tag available with that object to the device and, in so doing, activated the first sound source to the next destination. The same procedure was repeated for each activity. Data showed that both women were successful with the system and reached percentages of correct travels that were above or about 90.

Lancioni et al. (2009a) carried out a study with a 27-year-old woman who was in a wheelchair, had minimal residual vision, and was rated within the moderate intellectual disability range. The woman used a portable device with six keys. Five of them corresponded to as many destinations/activities and were covered with a small object that signaled the activity available at the related destination. Each of these keys was also encircled by small lights. As soon as the woman pressed one of the keys, (a) the sound source at the corresponding destination was activated and emitted verbal messages at intervals of 15 s, (b) the lights around the key switched off (and the key would no longer respond to any additional/erroneous pressure), and (c) the door of the room containing the destinations was marked with colored lights. The sixth key served to the woman to deactivate the sound source as soon as she arrived at the destination. Data showed that the percentage of correct travel was below 10 during the initial baseline, increased to a mean of about 75 during the first intervention phase, and dropped to 20 during the second baseline to increase to about 90 during the second intervention phase.

Visual (Light) Cues

Lancioni et al. (1996c) carried out the first study with the use of visual orientation cues. The main reasoning behind the use of visual cues was that they (a) may be as effective as auditory cues for persons with some levels of visual ability even when those levels are limited or minimal, (b) can be applied with persons who have auditory impairments, and (c) can minimize the amount of disturbance caused to individuals sharing the context in which those cues are employed (Lancioni et al. 1996c, 2007). The participants were two young men of 18 and 19 years of age who were rated within the profound intellectual disabilities range and presented with severe visual impairment. The system included a portable device for the selection of the destinations similar to that used by Lancioni et al. (1995a) and a variety of light sources used along the routes to the destinations. Each light box contained a coded radio receiver activated by a signal of the portable device, an electromagnetic generator for the proximity sensor of the portable device, and a battery. Two lamps were mounted on each box. Each lamp emitted approximately one flash per second. The cumulative intensity of two flashes was about 3 lux at a distance of 1 m. The selection of a destination through the portable device activated the first light box on the way to the destination. Once the participant was close to the box, the proximity sensor switched it off and activated the next/last one so that the participant could reach the destination. The participants' overall percentages of correct travels during the baseline phases were below 20. Their percentages during the intervention phases were close to 90 or above it.

Lancioni et al. (1998a) carried out two single-case studies with a 27-year-old woman and a 19-year-old man, respectively. In both studies, the aim was to promote activity and travel in persons who had the tendency to be passive and sedentary. The woman was diagnosed with blindness in one eye and highly reduced vision in the other, deafness, and profound intellectual disability. The procedural conditions were identical to those applied in the study by Lancioni et al. (1998b) except that the light cues replaced the sound sources. In essence, the participant found a Velcro tag (a token) to attach to the front panel of the portable device at the start of the session and at each activity. Pressing (attaching) this tag to the panel-switch activated the first light source of the first/next route programmed in the device. The man was diagnosed with low vision and profound intellectual disability. The procedural conditions applied with him involved the use of a portable device that worked on a time basis, that is, activated a new destination automatically after a preset interval from the man reaching the previous one had elapsed (see Lancioni et al. 1999a). In practice, when the participant reached a destination, a timer in the portable device switched on. At the end of a preset interval (i.e., a time estimated to be sufficient for the participant to carry out the activity available), the device automatically activated the first source to the next destination. The results of both studies were positive with the two participants developing effective orientation performance and reaching percentages of correct travels of approximately or above 90.

Lancioni et al. (2000b) used the orientation system with visual cues to help a 35-year-old woman to travel and carry out activities as a form of exercise that was intended to improve her general physical condition in addition to increasing her adaptive engagement. Both these goals were considered important because the woman tended to be passive and sedentary and was overweight. The woman, who was generally provided with two 30-min sessions in the morning and two 30-min sessions in the afternoon, learned to use the system and maintained its use over a relatively long period of time. The travel and activity (i.e., exercise) that the woman performed seemed to (a) have a positive effect on her ability to rise from a squatting position with reduced amount of help (i.e., suggesting an improvement in muscle condition), (b) promote a reduction in the excretion levels of urinary calcium and urinary hydroxyproline (i.e., suggesting positive effects on bone metabolism with possible long-term effects on bone mineral density), and (c) bring about a reduction in body weight independent of special diets (i.e., suggesting a beneficial impact in an area of concern with this participant and many other persons with intellectual and multiple disabilities, that is, excessive body weight).

Studies of Orientation Systems with Corrective Feedback

Orientation systems relying on corrective feedback (contrary to orientation systems with direction cues) are intended for persons with traveling initiative and relatively adequate spatial knowledge. They are designed to allow these individuals self-determination and freedom and, at the same time, to provide them with a form of assistance (i.e., a reliable help line) that would guarantee a successful outcome to their travel performance (Lancioni et al. 2007, 2009b). In practice, the system would not intervene at all on the participant's performance (thus avoiding any interference with his or her personal independence) as long as he or she follows the correct direction. It would, however, intervene with corrective feedback if the person takes an incorrect direction (i.e., a direction not contemplated within his or her route to the destination). The feedback would continue until the person finds the correct direction again. Only five studies were directed at assessing the use of this system (Lancioni and Mantini 1999; Lancioni et al. 1994a, 1995b, 1997a, 2000b). Those studies included a total of seven participants.

Lancioni et al. (1994a) carried out the first study aimed at developing this type of orientation system. Two men were involved as participants. One of them presented with blindness, motor impairment, and spatial disorientation but was not considered to have specific intellectual disability (i.e., he was described as a borderline case). The other man had a diagnosis of total blindness, deafness, and hemiplegia. Moreover, he presented a level of functioning seemingly compatible with a severe intellectual disability condition. Both participants had been involved in travel programs with the help of a mobile robot (see Introduction and Lancioni et al. 1993a, b). The orientation system developed for them consisted of three main parts, that is, a control unit, infrared light sources, and a portable device. The control unit served to regulate the other two components of the package and was on a desk in the orientation setting. The infrared light sources represented spatial reference points for the portable device and were at the destinations and along the routes to them. The portable device contained a microprocessor, light sensors to detect the signals of the infrared light sources, a radio receiver linking it to the control unit, a vibrator, and input keys. It was designed to perform two practical functions, that is, (a) providing vibratory feedback in case of direction errors and (b) allowing the participant to enter/activate the routes to the destinations. The first function was realized automatically through the activation of the aforementioned vibrator. The second function required the participants to use the keys available on the main (external) side of the device. Those keys were modified so that they could be readily discriminated by the participants. In practice, the keys had specific covers/tags attached to them with prominent configurations of different textures.

For each activity (travel to a destination), the participant started by collecting an object signal representing it. Then, he checked the tag attached to it, found the key of the device with the identical tag, pressed this key/tag, and started to walk. If he walked in the right direction, the device remained silent. If he strayed from the right direction, the device started providing vibratory feedback. At that point, the participant was to interrupt his walking and start turning around slowly until the vibration stopped (i.e., until he had recovered the right direction again). Once the vibration had ended, he could resume walking. Once he reached the destination, he would sit and carry out a useful (familiar) activity. Thereafter, he would collect a new object signal for the next activity and restart the sequence described above. The participants reached a preset learning criterion of six sessions without staff prompting/guidance after 24 and 19 intervention sessions, respectively. The sessions were 45 min long for both participants. The correct performance seemed to remain consistent through a second intervention phase following an intermediate baseline check.

Lancioni et al. (1997a) carried out a study with a 38-year-old woman who was diagnosed with total blindness and had serious (albeit unspecified) intellectual disability with a Vineland age equivalent of about 3 years on her daily living skills. She was eager to engage in simple activities but required some assistance in traveling from one activity destination to the next within her daily context. The orientation system developed for the participant included small boxes emitting ultrasonic waves, which marked the routes to the activity destinations, and a portable control device connected to earpieces. The portable device interacted with the aforementioned boxes and served to present verbal praise or a buzzer feedback through the earpieces. Each travel started with the woman taking an object signal indicating the activity to carry out and attaching the Velcro tag available with that object to the front panel (switch) of the portable device. This activated a destination and the emission of praise or buzzer feedback. In practice, she received a brief praise message at intervals of about 10 s as long as she maintained the right direction.

In case of wrong direction, a buzzer sound started. Upon hearing this sound, the woman was to turn until the sound stopped and then she was to resume her walking. The woman learned to use the system profitably. She required some level of supervisor's guidance during the initial period of the intervention, but she gradually became independent showing high percentages of correct travel performance.

Lancioni and Mantini (1999) worked with a 30-year-old woman who was totally blind in one eye and had a minimal residual vision in the other eye. The woman was also deaf and had a diagnosis of profound intellectual disability. The orientation system included (a) a variety of boxes emitting ultrasonic waves, such as those described above for the study by Lancioni et al. (1997a), and (b) a portable device combined with a feedback case. The procedural sequence that the woman was to follow for each activity was identical to that described for the study mentioned above. The functioning of the portable device was, however, different. It remained totally silent while the woman was walking within the route to the destination selected. It provided vibratory feedback in case of incorrect direction (i.e., if the woman was diverging of about 20° from the direction required). In the latter situation, she was to turn to her left, as cued by the position of the feedback case, until the vibration stopped. Then, she could resume her walking to the destination. Data showed that the woman's percentages of correct travel increased above 95. She displayed a mean of about two correction instances per travel occasion. The mean time required for each correction instance declined to about 10 s.

Discussion

Outcome of the Studies

The results reported by the studies reviewed were generally quite positive, thus suggesting that orientation technology may be a highly valuable resource within education and rehabilitation programs for persons with severe/profound intellectual and multiple disabilities. The first consideration one can make in relation to this general picture is largely methodological (research-related) and may amount to a cautionary note. This note originates from the fact that, although all the studies employed adequate experimental designs, (a) the overall number of participants involved was relatively small and (b) the experimental work was carried out by basically one research center. Obviously, this note does not intend to diminish the value of the findings but simply to pinpoint the need for independent replications to establish the generality of the findings and investigate issues of generalization (e.g., generalization across patients, across research and staff personnel, and across cultural contexts) (Kennedy 2005; Parker 2009; Ross and Kelly 2009).

The reasons for the positive results of the studies/programs employing direction cues may be found on the linearity of the orientation behavior required to the participants, the large amount of support provided by the technology, and the availability of carefully arranged motivational conditions (Lancioni et al. 2007, 2009b). The behavior of directing one's own attention to a sound or a light cue is largely available among persons with severe/profound and multiple disabilities. The behavior of reaching the source may also be often available or easily established. The presence of these skills was generally checked among the participants of the studies. Whenever the skills were missing and the person had great uncertainty, preliminary intervention conditions would be arranged for him or her. One such case (a man with Alzheimer's disease), for whom specific intervention conditions were arranged, was reported by Lancioni et al. (2011).

Regarding the support provided by the technology, one can underline that (a) two or more sound or light sources were often used within each travel route so as to avoid large distances between the person's position and the cue (i.e., distances that could prevent the person from orienting properly and remaining consistently oriented) and (b) the interval between cues was initially relatively small so as to avoid that the person could walk into a lost position in between cues. Obviously, the amount of support was typically smaller with persons who had higher orientation and travel abilities and could be reduced as the persons became more familiar with orientation and traveling performance (see below). Regarding the motivational conditions, it should be emphasized here that the studies ensured that each of the participants would receive forms of stimulation considered to be motivating (reinforcing) in relation to the travel or the activity carried out immediately after the travel (at the destination). Based on the characteristics of the participants, the stimulation available could be (a) exclusively social (e.g., praise and approval comments) produced by the sound sources at the destinations or by the staff members the participants met at the destinations or (b) edible (e.g., a small portion of favorite food) available underneath the activity material at the destination and at the end of the session in relation to the exchange of the tokens (see above) (e.g., Lancioni et al. 1998b, c, 1999a, 2000b; Lancioni et al. 2010a, b, 2011).

The positive results obtained in the studies/programs using orientation systems with corrective feedback may require some clarification. The high percentages of correct travels may reveal only one side of the systems' impact. Namely, they explain that the participants could use such a feedback to correct their direction and eventually reach the destinations independently. The side that the percentages do not reveal concerns the number of times that the participants were required to correct their direction during each travel and the total amount of time that they spent in correcting their direction and eventually reaching the destination. Two studies in particular may help to shed some light on this side of the story, which cannot be considered secondary given its practical and personal implications (i.e., Lancioni and Mantini 1999; Lancioni et al. 2007, 2009a, b). The first of the two, which was summarized above, included a woman with minimal residual vision who lost the correct direction a mean of about two times per travel route and corrected herself in about 10 s at each instance. The second study (Lancioni et al. 1995b) involved two women with total blindness who were exposed to two programs, one including an orientation system with auditory direction cues and the other including an orientation system with corrective feedback. The data showed that both programs promoted high percentages of correct travels. Yet there were large differences in the amount of time required to reach the destinations with the two systems. Specifically, using the system with corrective feedback could double the traveling time to the destinations. Although no specific data were provided as to the number of corrections needed within each travel route and the time needed for each correction, the suggestion is that both these values were higher than those reported in the study by Lancioni and Mantini (1999).

In light of the above, one might argue that the use of orientation systems with corrective feedback should be adopted (as a realistic and likely successful approach) when at least one of the following three conditions is met. First, the person (with or without residual vision) is fairly competent about his or her traveling space and is likely to make only few mistakes. Second, the person has a residual vision, which helps him or her walk without veering (i.e., without straying from a path) or with few veering instances, thus incurring relatively few direction errors and requiring only infrequent corrections (Millar 1999). Third, the person is totally blind and likely to veer but can rely on walls or other walking lines for much of the travel routes, with the consequence that the number of direction errors is automatically reduced (limited) (Guth and LaDuke 1994, 1995; Lancioni et al. 2007).

Implications of the Studies

The data reported seem to represent fairly encouraging and cohesive evidence as to the possibility of promoting orientation and mobility with persons with severe/profound and multiple disabilities (including persons with degenerative neurological syndromes such as Alzheimer's disease). The ability to travel independently (without extra burden on staff and caregivers in general) can provide them new opportunities within their environment with obviously positive implications. The basic opportunities pointed out (and realized) within the studies include (a) traveling to different rooms of a day center and interacting with different people as part of a social-occupational engagement, (b) reaching different work and home areas connected with one's own desires and needs, (c) carrying out a series of relevant activities distributed over different workrooms as part of a vocational program, and (d) carrying out activities and traveling across work and residential areas for extended periods of time as a form of physical exercise.

The realization of the aforementioned opportunities may largely modify or erase a stereotyped picture of persons with orientation and traveling problems that are confined to a specific room and provided with limited forms of engagement within a circumscribed space. Traveling to different rooms of a day center and delivering or picking up objects and meeting different staff people could be a viable and desirable occupational employment for a number of persons who can carry out small transport duties and enjoy social interaction (Lancioni et al. 2010a, 2011).

They would not need to have specific activity skills or to be able to manage the portable device to enter the new destinations. In fact, the staff members that they meet could (a) provide them with new material to transport and (b) concurrently enter (activate) the destinations to which that material should be delivered in their portable device (Gadler et al. 2009; Gitlin et al. 2008; Mausbach et al. 2008).

Using the orientation system for reaching different work and home areas connected with one's own desires and needs may be an objective for persons whose level of functioning is sufficiently high (i.e., persons who are able to monitor their desires and needs' general strength as well as the right time for their satisfaction) (Lancioni et al. 2008). Obviously, caregivers may intervene with requests connected to those (desire and need) issues so as to promote or delay their realization. The level of independence (freedom) of those persons would be determined by their ability to use the orientation cues or corrective feedback to travel efficiently as well as their ability to enter the destinations required in the portable device (Lancioni et al. 2008).

Using an orientation system to carry out a series of relevant activities distributed over different spaces/rooms as part of a vocational program may be a positive (and preferred) alternative to engaging in a few activities within a small space (Lancioni et al. 1999b). This vocational occupation would be fully functional for the context if the participants were to be totally independent throughout the occupation session. To this end (i.e., to promote full independence), the studies have assessed different forms of portable devices, which seem suitable for persons with different levels of ability, not excluding those at the lower end of the range. For example, one of the devices (suitable for fairly resourceful persons) has the key areas covered by small objects corresponding to the activities to be carried out at the destinations. The person needs to remove one of those objects to activate a specific destination (Lancioni et al. 2010b). Another type of device (used extensively with auditory as well as visual direction cues) consists of a box with a front panel serving as switch. A simple response such as attaching a Velcro tag to it activates the first/following destination of the sequence prearranged for the work session (e.g., Lancioni et al. 1997b, 1998a, b). A final type of device (suitable for persons with a low level of functioning who would have difficulties to reliably/consistently attach a Velcro tag to the switch panel) works on a time schedule. It activates a new destination after a preset interval of time has elapsed from the participant reaching the previous destination of the sequence (e.g., Lancioni et al. 1999a).

Using an orientation system to carry out extended activities and travel as a form of physical exercise may be considered a valuable (health-promoting) employment of the system. This type of employment would be viable only in situations in which the person can carry out a number of activities, can use the direction cues or corrective feedback properly, and can manage the portable device to activate the destinations independently. To facilitate the participants' performance concerning the last aspect of the sequence, one should choose the most suitable form of portable device out of those listed above (Lancioni et al. 1998a, 1999a, 2010b).

Practical Considerations on the Use of the Systems

In light of the data reported and of the considerations put forward above, one could easily hypothesize that orientation systems with direction cues would be much more frequently used than orientation systems with corrective feedback. While the latter systems remain a plausible and functional solution for a rather specific (and relatively advanced) group of people, the former systems with direction cues may be applied with a large variety of people showing a wide range of problems (Lancioni et al. 2007, 2009b).

An analysis of these more widely applicable systems with direction cues cannot simply be restricted to their possible benefits for the persons directly relying on them (as done through the review of the studies), but it may also need to include a basic evaluation of their implications for the educational or rehabilitation context as a whole. The most immediate implications one might discuss concern (a) their workability/practicality within the environment (i.e., the ease with which they can be used, their cost in terms of staff time, and the interference they can have with other people sharing the environment) and (b) their transportability/applicability and effectiveness across settings (i.e., their capacity to promote generalization of orientation skills across settings).

With regard to the first point, at least three considerations may be in order. First, sound sources or light boxes are battery-powered devices that can easily be arranged along the routes (i.e., on the walls or at the doors) conducting to the destinations as well as at the destinations. They are relatively small (e.g., 13 cm × 10 cm × 6 cm) and could also be made smaller through the use of new (upgraded) technical components (Bache and Derwent 2008; Baker and Moon 2008; Chantry and Dunford 2010; Reichle 2011; Johnson et al. 2009; Kagohara 2011). Thus, their physical presence can hardly create any difficulties for other persons in the context. Second, the time required to staff for preparing the technology for the participant (e.g., programming the sequence of destinations that he or she has to reach in the portable device and distributing the sources along the routes and at the destinations) is relatively small and may not need to be done on a daily basis. Third, the sound and visual cues emitted by the sources/boxes may easily interfere with other persons (staff and patients) sharing the environment with study participants. Given the nature of the cues, one cannot imagine of eliminating the disturbance. Efforts, however, can be made to reduce it to an acceptable level. To this end, studies have investigated the possibility of increasing the intervals between cues and have succeeded in maintaining high levels of correct travel performance with lower frequencies of cues (Lancioni et al. 1998d, 2001).

With regard to the second point, the first comment is that the technology is suited (given the small dimensions of the components involved and the fact that they are battery-powered) for being transported to and used in different settings. The possibility to transport the technology with ease is the basic requirement for using it to promote generalization of the participants' orientation and travel skills across settings (Cherrier et al. 2001; Kazdin 2001). Indeed, a number of the studies reviewed above have assessed the generalization aspect and have reported highly positive results in this area (Lancioni et al. 1995a, 1996c, 1998c, 2009a, 2010b). These findings are highly relevant to justify the use of orientation technology with persons with severe/profound and multiple disabilities. Other attempts to teach them the orientation and travel skills (e.g., backward-chaining strategies; see Introduction) would be very costly in terms of staff time and relatively uncertain as to the general outcome. Moreover, they could not ensure that the skill trained would easily generalize to new environments (Brooks et al. 1999; Kazdin 2001; Lancioni et al. 2011; Provencher et al. 2008).

Conclusions

The studies reviewed in this chapter underline the relevance of orientation systems for promoting independent travel and activity in persons with severe/profound and multiple disabilities. Systems based on corrective feedback may be realistically used only with persons who have a relatively advanced notion of traveling and space and can avoid frequent direction errors. Systems based on direction cues can be used very widely. The decision to rely on auditory or visual cues is to be determined on the person's characteristics. The same characteristics would also determine which type of portable device should be adopted, that is, (a) a portable device where the participant is to select each activity/destination directly, (b) a portable device where the participant is entering the destinations according to the sequence preset by the supervisor, or (c) a portable device where the selection of destinations is automatically performed (i.e., it is time-based). Successful use of the system within the learning setting is likely to generalize across new settings with important practical implications.

New research initiatives in the area could focus on several methodological and practical questions. First, additional participants should be involved in research programs with both systems to determine the generality of the data reported. Moreover, the research should be carried out by different experimenters and in different geographical and national contexts to isolate any possible influence of environmental and cultural variables (Kennedy 2005; Parker 2009). Second, special research attention may be devoted to an emerging group of persons with special needs, that is, persons with neurodegenerative diseases such as the Alzheimer's disease. Third, efforts may be made to upgrade the technology so as to reduce the dimensions of the different components and make their programming easier and less time costly. The new technology may also be more versatile so that its functioning could be easily tailored to the characteristics of the persons involved. Fourth, preference assessments might be carried out to determine whether the participants enjoy activity and traveling supported by the orientation devices more than other activity arrangements (Lancioni et al. 1999b).

References

Algozzine, B., Browder, D., Karvonen, M., Test, D. W., & Wood, W. M. (2001). Effects of interventions to promote self-determination for individuals with disabilities. *Review of Educational Research, 71*, 219–277.

Bache, J., & Derwent, G. (2008). Access to computer-based leisure for individuals with profound disabilities. *NeuroRehabilitation, 23*, 343–350.

Baker, P. M., & Moon, N. W. (2008). Wireless technologies and accessibility for people with disabilities: Findings from a policy research instrument. *Assistive Technology, 20*, 149–156.

Baldwin, D. (2003). Wayfinding technology: A road map to the future. *Journal of Visual Impairment and Blindness, 97*, 612–620.

Brooks, B. M., McNeil, J. E., Rose, F. D., Greenwood, R. J., Attree, E. A., & Leadbetter, A. G. (1999). Route learning in a case of amnesia: A preliminary investigation into the efficacy of training in a virtual environment. *Neuropsychological Rehabilitation, 9*, 63–76.

Chantry, J., & Dunford, C. (2010). How do computer assistive technologies enhance participation in childhood occupations for children with multiple and complex disabilities: A review of the current literature. *British Journal of Occupational Therapy, 73*, 351–365.

Cherrier, M. M., Mendez, M., & Perryman, K. (2001). Route learning performance in Alzheimer disease patients. *Neuropsychiatry, Neuropsychology, and Behavioral Neurology, 14*, 159–168.

Draheim, C. C., Williams, D. P., & McCubbin, J. A. (2002). Prevalence of physical inactivity and recommended physical activity in community-based adults with mental retardation. *Mental Retardation, 40*, 436–444.

Gadler, E., Grassi, A., & Riva, G. (2009). A rehabilitation protocol for empowering spatial orientation in MCI: A pilot study. *Annual Review of CyberTherapy and Telemedicine, 7*, 234–236.

Gibson, M. C., MacLean, J., Borrie, M., & Geiger, J. (2004). Orientation behaviors in residents relocated to a redesigned dementia care unit. *American Journal of Alzheimer's Disease and Other Dementias, 19*, 45–49.

Gitlin, L. N., Winter, L., Burke, J., Chernett, N., Dennis, M. P., & Hauck, W. W. (2008). Tailored activities to manage neuropsychiatric behaviors in persons with dementia and reduce caregiver burden: A randomized pilot study. *The American Journal of Geriatric Psychiatry, 16*, 229–239.

Guth, D., & LaDuke, R. (1994). The veering tendency of blind pedestrians: An analysis of the problem and literature review. *Journal of Visual Impairment and Blindness, 88*, 391–400.

Guth, D., & LaDuke, R. (1995). Veering by blind pedestrians: Individual differences and their implications for instruction. *Journal of Visual Impairment and Blindness, 89*, 28–37.

Higgerty, M. J., & Williams, A. C. (2005). Orientation and mobility training using small groups. *Journal of Visual Impairment and Blindness, 99*, 755–764.

Jerome, J., Frantino, E. P., & Sturmey, P. (2007). The effects of errorless learning and backward chaining on the acquisition of Internet skills in adults with developmental disabilities. *Journal of Applied Behavior Analysis, 40*, 185–189.

Joffee, E. (1995). Approaches to teaching orientation and mobility. In K. M. Huebner, J. G. Prickett, T. R. Welch, & E. Joffee (Eds.), *Hand in hand: Essentials of communication and orientation and mobility for your students who are deaf-blind* (pp. 575–611). New York: AFB Press.

Joffee, E., & Rikhye, C. H. (1991). Orientation and mobility for students with severe visual and multiple impairments: A new perspective. *Journal of Visual Impairment and Blindness, 85*, 211–216.

Johnson, K. L., Bamer, A. M., & Amtmann, D. (2009). Use of cognitive aids and other assistive technology by individuals with multiple sclerosis. *Disability and Rehabilitation: Assistive Technology, 4*, 1–8.

Kagohara, D. M. (2011). Three students with developmental disabilities learn to operate an iPod to access age-appropriate entertainment videos. *Journal of Behavioral Education, 20*, 33–43.

Karvonen, M., Test, D. W., Wood, W. M., Browder, D., & Algozzine, B. (2004). Putting self-determination into practice. *Exceptional Children, 71*, 23–41.

Kazdin, A. E. (2001). *Behavior modification in applied settings* (6th ed.). New York: Wadsworth.

Kennedy, C. (2005). *Single case designs for educational research*. New York: Allyn & Bacon.

Konrad, M., Fowler, C. H., Walker, A. R., Test, D. W., & Wood, W. M. (2007). Effects of self-determination interventions on the academic skills of students with learning disabilities. *Learning Disability Quarterly, 30*, 89–113.

Lachapelle, Y., Wehmeyer, M. L., Haelewyck, M. C., Courbois, Y., Keith, K. D., Schalock, R., Verdugo, M. A., & Walsh, P. N. (2005). The relationship between quality of life and self-determination: An international study. *Journal of Intellectual Disability Research, 49*, 740–744.

Lancioni, G. E., Bellini, D., & Oliva, D. (1993a). A robot to provide multihandicapped blind persons with physical guidance and activity choices. *Journal of Developmental and Physical Disabilities, 5*, 337–348.

Lancioni, G. E., Bellini, D., & Oliva, D. (1993b). Building choice opportunities within a robot-assisted occupational program: A case study. *Behavioral Residential Treatment, 8*, 219–226.

Lancioni, G. E., Boelens, H., Oliva, D., & Bracalente, S. (1996a). Enabling blind persons with severe or profound mental retardation to operate an acoustic orientation system independently. *Behavioral Interventions, 11*, 207–215.

Lancioni, G. E., Campodonico, F., & Mantini, M. (2001). Supporting independent indoor travel of people with blindness and intellectual disability with reduced frequencies of auditory cues. *Perceptual and Motor Skills, 92*, 83–88.

Lancioni, G. E., Gigante, A., O'Reilly, M. F., & Oliva, D. (2000a). Evaluating mild physical exercise with two persons with profound multiple disabilities. *Journal of Visual Impairment and Blindness, 94*, 461–465.

Lancioni, G. E., Gigante, A., O'Reilly, M. F., Oliva, D., & Montironi, L. (2000b). Indoor travel and simple tasks as physical exercise for people with profound multiple disabilities. *Perceptual and Motor Skills, 91*, 211–216.

Lancioni, G. E., & Mantini, M. (1998). Two women with multiple disabilities sharing an acoustic orientation system and traveling together to indoor destinations. *Perceptual and Motor Skills, 87*, 1192–1194.

Lancioni, G. E., & Mantini, M. (1999). A corrective-feedback system for helping a person with multiple disabilities during indoor travel. *Perceptual and Motor Skills, 88*, 1291–1295.

Lancioni, G. E., Mantini, M., Cognini, I., & Pirani, P. (1998a). Facilitating ambulation and activity in persons with profound multiple disabilities through a visual orientation system. *Behavioral Interventions, 13*, 123–133.

Lancioni, G. E., Mantini, M., O'Reilly, M. F., & Oliva, D. (1999a). An adapted acoustic orientation system for promoting independent indoor travel and activity in persons with profound multiple disabilities. *Journal of Developmental and Physical Disabilities, 11*, 35–46.

Lancioni, G. E., & Oliva, D. (1999). Using an orientation system for indoor travel and activity with persons with multiple disabilities. *Disability and Rehabilitation, 21*, 124–127.

Lancioni, G. E., Oliva, D., & Bracalente, S. (1994a). An electronic guidance system for multihandicapped blind persons: Evaluating its effectiveness and likableness. *Behavioral Interventions, 9*, 93–103.

Lancioni, G. E., Oliva, D., & Bracalente, S. (1995a). An acoustic orientation system to promote independent indoor travel in blind persons with severe mental retardation. *Perceptual and Motor Skills, 80*, 747–754.

Lancioni, G. E., Oliva, D., & Bracalente, S. (1995b). Comparison of two orientation systems for indoor travel of blind persons with mental retardation. *Perceptual and Motor Skills, 81*, 643–650.

Lancioni, G. E., Oliva, D., & Bracalente, S. (1998c). A portable control device for promoting independent indoor travel by persons with severe multiple disabilities. *Journal of Visual Impairment & Blindness, 92*, 63–70.

Lancioni, G. E., Oliva, D., Bracalente, S., & ten Hoopen, G. (1996b). Use of an acoustic orientation system for indoor travel with a spatially disabled blind man. *Journal of Visual Impairment & Blindness, 90*, 36–42.

Lancioni, G. E., Oliva, D., & Gnocchini, F. (1996c). A visual orientation system for promoting indoor travel in persons with profound developmental disabilities and visual impairment. *Perceptual and Motor Skills, 83*, 619–626.

Lancioni, G. E., Oliva, D., & Gnocchini, F. (1998d). Enhancing independent indoor travel and activity in a woman with multiple disabilities through special technology. *International Journal of Rehabilitation Research, 21*, 409–413.

Lancioni, G. E., Oliva, D., Serenelli, S., & Pirani, P. (1997a). An unobtrusive system for helping a person with blindness and intellectual disability travel in indoor areas. *Perceptual and Motor Skills, 85*, 1431–1434.

Lancioni, G. E., Oliva, D., & Signorino, M. (1994b). Promoting ambulation and object manipulation in persons with multiple handicaps through the use of a robot. *Perceptual and Motor Skills, 79*, 843–848.

Lancioni, G. E., Oliva, D., & Ten Hoopen, G. (1997b). Spoken messages as auditory cues for orientation in promoting indoor travel and activity by persons with multiple disabilities. *Perceptual and Motor Skills, 85*, 403–410.

Lancioni, G. E., O'Reilly, M. F., & Mantini, M. (1999b). Activity arrangements with or without mobility and performance of persons with multiple disabilities over long sessions. *Irish Journal of Psychology, 20*, 124–135.

Lancioni, G. E., O'Reilly, M. F., Oliva, D., & Bracalente, S. (1998b). Guiding a person with blindness and intellectual disability in indoor travel with fewer auditory cues. *Journal of Visual Impairment & Blindness, 92*, 609–614.

Lancioni, G. E., O'Reilly, M. F., Singh, N. N., Sigafoos, J., Campodonico, F., & Oliva, D. (2009a). A wheelchair user with visual and intellectual disabilities managing simple orientation technology for indoor travel. *Journal of Visual Impairment and Blindness, 103*, 308–313.

Lancioni, G. E., O'Reilly, M. F., Singh, N. N., Sigafoos, J., & Oliva, D. (2009b). Orientation technology for indoor travel by persons with multiple disabilities. *Cognitive Processing, 10*(Suppl. 2), S244–S246.

Lancioni, G. E., O'Reilly, M. F., Singh, N. N., Sigafoos, J., Oliva, D., Bracalente, S., & Montironi, G. (2007). Orientation systems to support indoor travel by persons with multiple disabilities: Technical aspects and application issues. *Technology and Disability, 19*, 1–6.

Lancioni, G. E., Perilli, V., Singh, N. N., O'Reilly, M. F., Sigafoos, J., Bosco, A., De Caro, M. F., Cassano, G., Pinto, K., & Minervini, M. (2011). Persons with mild or moderate Alzheimer's disease use a basic orientation technology to travel to different rooms within a day center. *Research in Developmental Disabilities, 32*, 1985–1991.

Lancioni, G. E., Singh, N. N., O'Reilly, M. F., Sigafoos, J., Alberti, G., Scigliuzzo, F., Signorino, M., Oliva, D., Smaldone, A., & La Martire, M. L. (2010a). Persons with multiple disabilities use orientation technology to find room entrances during indoor traveling. *Research in Developmental Disabilities, 31*, 1577–1584.

Lancioni, G. E., Singh, N. N., O'Reilly, M. F., Sigafoos, J., Campodonico, F., & Oliva, D. (2008). Self-management of orientation technology and auditory cues for indoor travel by two persons with multiple disabilities. *Journal of Developmental and Physical Disabilities, 20*, 129–138.

Lancioni, G. E., Singh, N. N., O'Reilly, M. F., Sigafoos, J., Campodonico, F., & Oliva, D. (2010b). Two persons with multiple disabilities use orientation technology with auditory cues to manage simple indoor traveling. *Research in Developmental Disabilities, 31*, 397–402.

Marquardt, G., & Schmieg, P. (2009). Dementia-friendly architecture: Environments that facilitate wayfinding in nursing homes. *American Journal of Alzheimer's Disease and Other Dementias, 24*, 333–340.

Martelli, M. F., Nicholson, K., & Zasler, N. D. (2008). Skill reacquisition after acquired brain injury: A holistic habit retraining model of neurorehabilitation. *NeuroRehabilitation, 23*, 115–126.

Martinsen, H., Tellevik, J. M., Elmerskog, B., & StorlilØkken, M. (2007). Mental effort in mobility route learning. *Journal of Visual Impairment and Blindness, 101*, 327–338.

Mausbach, B. T., Coon, D. W., Patterson, T. L., & Grant, I. (2008). Engagement in activities is associated with affective arousal in Alzheimer's caregivers: A preliminary examination of the temporal relations between activity and affect. *Behavior Therapy, 39*, 366–374.

McGilton, K. S., Rivera, T. M., & Dawson, P. (2003). Can we help persons with dementia find their way in a new environment? *Aging & Mental Health, 7*, 363–371.

Millar, S. (1999). Veering re-visited: Noise and posture cues in walking without sight. *Perception, 28*, 765–780.

Parker, A. T. (2009). Orientation and mobility with persons who are deaf-blind: An initial examination of single-subject-design research. *Journal of Visual Impairment and Blindness, 103*, 372–377.

Petry, K., Maes, B., & Vlaskamp, C. (2005). Domains of quality of life of people with profound multiple disabilities: The perspective of parents and direct support staff. *Journal of Applied Research in Intellectual Disabilities, 18*, 35–46.

Petry, K., Maes, B., & Vlaskamp, C. (2009). Measuring the quality of life of people with profound multiple disabilities using the QOL-PMD: First results. *Research in Developmental Disabilities, 30*, 1394–1405.

Provencher, V., Bier, N., Audet, T., & Gagnon, L. (2008). Errorless-based techniques can improve route finding in early Alzheimer's disease: A case study. *American Journal of Alzheimer's Disease and Other Dementias, 23*, 47–56.

Rainville, C., Passini, R., & Marchand, N. (2001). A multiple case study of wayfinding in dementia of the Alzheimer type: Decision making. *Aging Neuropsychology and Cognition, 8*, 54–71.

Reichle, J. (2011). Evaluating assistive technology in the education of persons with severe disabilities. *Journal of Behavioral Education, 20*, 77–85.

Ross, D. A., & Kelly, G. W. (2009). Filling the gaps for indoor wayfinding. *Journal of Visual Impairment and Blindness, 103*, 229–234.

Uslan, M. (1976). Teaching basic ward layout to the severely retarded blind: An auditory approach. *The New Outlook for the Blind, 70*, 401–402.

Uslan, M., Malone, S., & De L'Aune, W. (1983). Teaching route travel to multiply handicapped blind adults: An auditory approach. *Journal of Visual Impairment and Blindness, 77*, 18–20.

Uslan, M., Russell, I., & Weiner, C. (1988). A "musical pathway" for spatially disoriented blind residents of a skilled nursing facility. *Journal of Visual Impairment and Blindness, 82*, 21–24.

Chapter 6
Technology-Based Approaches for Promoting Ambulation

Abstract This chapter provides an overview of studies using technology-based approaches to promote ambulation in participants with intellectual disabilities and motor delays (i.e., children with Down syndrome) or with multiple disabilities (i.e., combinations of intellectual and neuromotor disabilities or of intellectual, neuromotor, and sensory disabilities). The most popular technology-based approach consists of the use of treadmills. A second technology-based approach combines the use of walker devices with microswitches. The microswitches allow the monitoring of the person's stepping responses and the automatic delivery of brief periods of preferred stimulation contingent on those responses. A third technology-based approach, representing an early attempt to develop technological support for ambulation, consists of the use of a mobile robot. This chapter provides an overview of the different approaches by summarizing the studies using them, their procedural conditions, their differences in emphasis and aims, and their outcomes. This chapter also provides (a) a discussion of the results obtained with the different approaches and their implications in terms of applicability, practicality, and suitability of the approaches within education (rehabilitation) contexts and (b) a brief presentation of some relevant issues for future research in the area.

Introduction

Walking (or ambulation) is a critical skill with a multitude of practical and social implications. Indeed, walking can be instrumental in allowing a person to reach different target places, to get involved in different activities, and to meet others (Hayakawa and Kobayashi 2011; Lancioni et al. 2009b; Schmidt et al. 2007). Walking is also a strategy that a person may use to promote his or her overall fitness and health condition (Cirignano et al. 2010; Lancioni et al. 2000a, b; Lee et al. 2010; Lotan et al. 2004a). While walking and the fulfillment of all its functions appear very natural (and unfold in a largely predictable manner) in typically developing persons, a different

G.E. Lancioni et al., *Assistive Technology: Interventions for Individuals with Severe/Profound and Multiple Disabilities*, Autism and Child Psychopathology Series, DOI 10.1007/978-1-4614-4229-5_6,

picture often emerges for persons with developmental disabilities (Cernak et al. 2008; Cherng et al. 2007; Chia et al. 2010; Katz-Leurer et al. 2010).

A certain group of persons with developmental disabilities may present with very extensive neuromotor impairment that prevents them from achieving any functional walking skills and confines them to the use of wheelchairs or similar means (Lancioni et al. 2009a; Liso 2010; Simard-Tremblay et al. 2010). A second group of these persons may also present with neuromotor impairment, but the level and extensiveness of this impairment may be more contained and allow them to achieve some form of functional walking (Maher et al. 2011; Whittingham et al. 2010). Such walking may fail to be fluent and require some level of support or the use of aids such as crutches and orthoses (Lancioni et al. 2009b; Nolan et al. 2010; Van Gestel et al. 2008).

The most common intervention approach employed to improve the condition of children with cerebral palsy and persons with motor and intellectual disabilities in general (and possibly foster some level of walking with them) has relied on the neurodevelopmental method (Bar-Haim et al. 2006; Begnoche and Pitetti 2007; Day et al. 2004; Ketelaar et al. 2001; Tsorlakis et al. 2004). The neurodevelopmental method is largely based on the conceptual model devised by the Bobaths (see Bobath 1980; Bobath and Bobath 1984). This model emphasizes the importance of promoting normal muscle activity as a basis for improving posture and the development of postural control as the foundation for movement. Rehabilitation is considered a process whereby the person gains motor abilities with the help of the therapist's facilitation and inhibition procedures. Facilitation refers to the use of sensory information (i.e., verbal directions and tactile cues/guidance) to promote and support weak posture or movement components. Inhibition, by contrast, refers to the use of the aforementioned types of information for reducing posture or movement components that are abnormal and interfere with the performance of the correct ones (Cherng et al. 2007; Ketelaar et al. 2001; Tsorlakis et al. 2004). Within this model, the use of compensation (i.e., increased role of the more functional side to make up for the less functional side) is viewed as unnecessary and dangerous. Similarly, the use of muscle strengthening exercises is viewed as an inadequate approach that is likely to increase spasticity and promote abnormal movement patterns.

The influence of the neurodevelopmental method, albeit still considerable, has been declining steadily over the last 10–15 years, due to (a) the evidence countering the method's early interpretation of the reflexes and their functions, (b) demonstrations that exercises for strengthening legs' muscles are effective in achieving such a goal and improving the muscles' functional use without increasing spasticity, (c) lack of specific scientific evidence attesting that the neurodevelopmental method produces rehabilitation effects significantly greater than other intervention methods, and (d) increasing attention and data concerning the training and exercise approach (Anttila et al. 2008; Blundell et al. 2003; Day et al. 2004; Hamed and Abd-elwahab 2011; Ketelaar et al. 2001; Kollen et al. 2009).

This last approach, which is based on the notion of experience-dependent plasticity, suggests that the way to improve a person's ambulatory behavior is to allow that person to successfully practice such behavior (Begnoche and Pitetti 2007; Kollen et al. 2009). The most popular technology-based approach developed in line with this new perspective is the one that relies on the use of treadmills generally combined with partial body weight support (Accivatti et al. 2006; Damiano and DeJong 2009; Dannemiller et al. 2005; DeJong et al. 2005; Sanders et al. 2005; Zwicker and Mayson 2010). The strategy of supporting the person's body weight (e.g., through a harness) may be essential to facilitate his or her stepping responses particularly when the level of motor impairment is more severe or the person's (child's) motor condition is largely immature (Angulo-Barroso et al. 2008a, b; Beard et al. 2005; Provost et al. 2007; Schindl et al. 2000). Orthopedic shoes and orthoses can be kept in use (i.e., for those persons who are accustomed to them) (Schindl et al. 2000; Willoughby et al. 2010). A second technology-based approach, in line with the same perspective, is the one that combines the use of walker devices with microswitches. The walkers can be equipped with supporting features that promote postural control and partial weight lifting. The microswitches allow the monitoring of the participant's stepping responses and the automatic delivery of brief periods of preferred environmental stimulation contingent on those responses (Lancioni et al. 2005a, 2007a). A third technology-based approach, which might be briefly presented here as one of the early attempts to resort to technological support in promoting ambulation, concerns the use of a mobile robot (Lancioni et al. 1993a, b, 1997).

This chapter is directed at examining the aforementioned technology-based approaches by providing an overview of the studies using those approaches to promote ambulation in participants with intellectual disabilities and motor delays (i.e., children with Down syndrome) or with multiple disabilities (i.e., combinations of intellectual and neuromotor disabilities or of intellectual, neuromotor, and sensory disabilities). The overview (summary) of the studies is aimed at providing an illustration of the specific procedural conditions (and specific emphasis and aims) characterizing the single approaches and a general picture of the outcomes reported. This chapter also provides (a) a discussion of those outcomes and their implications in terms of applicability, practicality, and suitability of the approaches within education (rehabilitation) contexts and (b) a brief presentation of some relevant issues for future research in the area.

Studies Reporting the Use of a Robot

As suggested above, the use of a mobile robot as a support system for persons with multiple disabilities was an early attempt to employ technology for promoting ambulation (Lancioni et al. 1989, 1993a). The first point to clarify about this approach is that it was aimed at persons who could walk with support. The second consideration is that the reasoning behind the studies was not specifically focused on improving the persons' walking skills per se. Rather, it was to ensure that they could practice walking and make this useful to reach activity destinations and engage in some form of physical exercise (countering their excessive sedentariness). Four studies may be listed here as examples of this approach providing a view of its application and impact (Lancioni et al. 1993b, 1994, 1997, 2000a).

Lancioni et al. (1993b) carried out a study with two participants (a man and a woman) of 18 and 19 years of age, respectively. The man was totally blind and deaf and was affected by hemiplegia with poor balance and uncertain ambulatory behavior. He was able to carry out a variety of simple activities and communicated through gestures, mimicry, and some basic fingerspelling. The woman also was blind, but she had typical hearing and could express herself verbally. She presented with hemiplegia, needed physical support for walking, and was overweight. Like the man, she could engage in a variety of small vocational activities within her daily context. The setting for the robot-assisted program included three connecting rooms. The robot was 52 cm wide and 106 cm high. It had large handles at the two main sides of it. One handle was just beneath a large keyboard (with keys covered by object replicas; see below). The participants could comfortably hold onto the handles to receive physical support and guidance to the activity destinations. It moved by means of four driving wheels connected to two independent battery-powered engines. The speed was programmable and was regulated at 0.27 m/s for the man and 0.19 m/s for the woman. Withdrawal of the participant's hands from the handle or an obstacle on the way made the robot stop its movement.

The robot was used in combination with a supply device. At the start of an ambulation and activity session, the participants were to choose between two object signals (i.e., small object replicas representing two different activities) at the supply device. The choice of one object (activity) was to be followed by the activation (pressing) of the key of the robot covered by an object replica matching the one that they had selected from the supply device. This made the robot select the route to the related activity destination out of the routes that had been programmed into its memory. The robot started moving as the participant took hold of the handle beneath the keyboard, thus breaking the light beam of optic sensors located there. When the robot reached the activity destination, the sensors at the handle that the participant had used went off and the sensors at the other handle switched on. Once the participants had carried out the activity, they could take hold of the robot's handle closer to them (the only one with the sensors "on"). This triggered the robot to travel the route back to the supply device where the sequence restarted. Both participants were able to use the robot successfully to reach the activity destinations from the supply device and return to the supply device to operate new activity choices. This allowed them to maintain a combination of travel and constructive occupational engagement through the sessions, which lasted up to 45 min.

Lancioni et al. (1994) used the same mobile robot described above with a man and a woman of 23 and 18 years of age, respectively. The man was rated in the profound range of intellectual disability and presented with total blindness, deafness, spastic tetraparesis, and a form of ataxia making his balance very precarious. When provided with support, he could walk slowly but without apparent difficulties. The woman was diagnosed with total blindness, profound intellectual disability, spastic tetraparesis with severe scoliosis, and pelvic asymmetry. She could walk in small steps when provided with adequate support. The program was aimed at promoting ambulation and activity. The participants were to transport objects through an adapted shirt, which was provided with specially arranged pockets. After receiving the objects, the participants would take hold of the robot's handle and walk behind the robot until reaching a couch. At that point, they would sit on the couch and put away the objects. The participants were allowed to sit on the couch for 1–3 min before starting the next move to the next destination/couch where to sit and put away the objects. Both participants managed a fairly successful performance in terms of activity and ambulation. Their average walking time was between 20 and 22 min per session. Staff personnel interviewed about the participants' appearance and behavior during different daily conditions expressed positive views of the participants' performance during the sessions with the robot.

Lancioni et al. (1997) replicated and extended the results of the previous Lancioni et al.'s (1994) study with two men of 24 and 18 years of age, respectively. Both men were diagnosed with blindness and profound intellectual disabilities. They also presented with severe auditory impairment and extensive neuromotor disabilities that prevented them from walking without support. As in the previous studies, the aim was to promote the participants' ambulation and occupational engagement. The participants were to transport objects and put them away once they had reached a couch where they would sit for 2–3 min and receive vibratory (preferred) stimulation. Three measures were recorded during the study, that is, the frequency of correct activities (i.e., transporting and putting away objects independently), the number of minutes that the participants walked independently, and staff's judgments of the participants' tiredness on the basis of videotaped sequences. Data showed that the participants performed most of the activities correctly and reached a mean time of over 20 min of independent walking per session by the end of the first intervention phase. Given their successful performance and lack of any detectable signs of tiredness, the number of activities was gradually increased so that by the end of the second intervention period, they reached a mean walking time per session of about 30 min. This increase did not interfere with the high level of correct (independent) performance. No evaluation was carried out of any specific improvements in the participants' walking. The view was that the walking experience (practice) would be likely to have beneficial effects on muscle strength and coordination and could also reduce the risks associated with the sedentary lifestyles that these persons are accustomed to have (Cirignano et al. 2010; Lancioni et al. 2000a, b; Lee et al. 2010; Lotan et al. 2004a). The walking was also thought to have a positive impact on the participants' social image, in line with the support for ambulation and activity expressed by the staff in the previous study (Lancioni et al. 2004).

Studies Reporting the Use of a Treadmill

The studies using the treadmill approach were mostly characterized by (a) the inclusion of children as participants, (b) the use of partial body weight support to help them respond appropriately and avoid rapid tiredness, and (c) the emphasis on

Table 6.1 Studies using treadmill intervention and involving participants with Down syndrome, cerebral palsy, and Rett syndrome

Studies	Participants	Age	Conditions
Down syndrome			
Ulrich et al. (2001)	30	10 months	Treadmill intervention versus control
Wu et al. (2007)	45	10 months	Higher-intensity-personalized treadmill protocol versus lower-intensity-generalized treadmill protocol versus control
Ulrich et al. (2008)	30	10 months	Higher-intensity-personalized treadmill protocol versus lower-intensity-generalized treadmill protocol
Angulo-Barroso et al. (2008a)	30[a]	10 months	Higher-intensity-personalized treadmill protocol versus lower-intensity-generalized treadmill protocol
Angulo-Barroso et al. (2008b)	30[a]	10 months	Higher-intensity-personalized treadmill protocol versus lower-intensity-generalized treadmill protocol
Wu et al. (2008)	30[a]	10 months	Higher-intensity-personalized treadmill protocol versus lower-intensity-generalized treadmill protocol
Looper and Ulrich (2010)	22	10 months	Treadmill intervention plus orthosis versus treadmill intervention
Cerebral palsy and Rett syndrome			
Schindl et al. (2000)	10	6–18 years	Treadmill intervention
Dodd and Foley (2007)	14	5–15 years	Treadmill intervention versus control
Borggraefe et al. (2008)	1	6 years	Treadmill intervention
Willoughby et al. (2010)	26	5–18 years	Treadmill intervention versus overground walking practice
Lotan et al. (2004b)	4	8.5–11 years	Treadmill intervention

[a]These same participants are involved in these studies

walking practice and exercise with the aim of improving the whole gait cycle and eventually promoting walking skills (Accivatti et al. 2006; Begnoche and Pitetti 2007; Damiano and DeJong 2009; Zwicker and Mayson 2010). Of the numerous studies that have been conducted with the use of treadmills, only 12 are referred to in this chapter. Those 12 studies were selected because they included participants with apparent intellectual and communication disabilities in addition to their motor impairment or delay. Seven of the 12 studies were concerned with infants and young children with Down syndrome (Angulo-Barroso et al. 2008a, b; Looper and Ulrich 2010; Ulrich et al. 2001, 2008; Wu et al. 2007, 2008). The other five studies included children with cerebral palsy or Rett syndrome (Borggraefe et al. 2008; Dodd and Foley 2007; Lotan et al. 2004b; Schindl et al. 2000; Willoughby et al. 2010). Table 6.1 lists all the aforementioned studies.

Participants with Down Syndrome

The age of the children at the beginning of the studies was mostly around 10 months. The two main criteria used for their inclusion in the studies were (a) the ability to produce six steps per minute while supported on the treadmill or (b) the ability to sit independently for 30 s. Body weight support was obtained via direct intervention of parents and therapists rather than through a harness.

Ulrich et al. (2001) assessed the impact of early treadmill intervention on the achievement of raising self to stand, walking with help, and walking independently. The study involved the participation of 30 children whose age at the start of the study averaged 307 days. The children were divided into two groups. One group received treadmill intervention and biweekly pediatric physical therapy. The other group received only biweekly pediatric physical therapy. The first group had custom-engineered treadmills placed at their homes, and parents were instructed to position them on the treadmills, hold them upright so their feet were flat on the treadmill belt, and carry out the intervention (i.e., ensure that they produced stepping responses in relation to the movement of the treadmill belt) 5 days a week. The intervention was programmed to last 8 min per day. Initially, the children would be held on the treadmill per intervals of 1 min followed by 1-min rest periods. Gradually, the intervals on the treadmill were extended up to the point that they covered the 8-min period with no rest interruptions. The children receiving treadmill intervention reached each of the three milestones on which measurements were made (i.e., rising to stand, walking with help, and walking independently) in a shorter amount of time from entering the program than the control children. Specifically, they reached (a) rising to stand after a mean of 134 days, (b) walking with help after a mean of 166 days, and (c) walking independently after a mean of 300 days. The control children reached the same milestones after 194, 240, and 401 days, respectively. The differences on the last two milestones (i.e., walking with help and walking independently) were statistically significant.

Wu et al. (2007) evaluated the impact of different intensities of treadmill intervention on the acquisition of walking skills and on the subsequent development of gait patterns. Their hypotheses were that (a) children who received treadmill intervention would walk earlier and present a more advanced gait pattern (e.g., faster walking speed or longer strides) than children who did not receive such intervention and (b) children receiving a higher-intensity-individualized intervention protocol would have better results than those receiving a lower-intensity-generalized intervention protocol. The treadmill speed was set at 0.18 m/s. Higher-intensity-individualized intervention involved a rise in demands tailored to individual progress. The rise concerned increases in the treadmill speed (which reached about 0.22 m/s), extensions in the daily use of the treadmill (which reached about 9 min), and application of little weights to the children's ankles (which exceeded 300 g). The intervention protocols were maintained until the children reached the criterion of walking onset (i.e., three independent steps performed successively overground). The walking onset criterion was achieved at 23.9 months of age by the 15 children who constituted the control group (i.e., who had no treadmill intervention), at 21.4 months of age by the 14 children who received the lower-intensity-generalized intervention protocol, and at 19.2 months of age by the 16 children who received the higher-intensity-individualized intervention protocol. Statistical analyses indicated that the differences were significant only between the first and the third group of children. In line with the walking onset results, gait data indicated that the stride length of the children who received the higher-intensity-individualized intervention protocol was significantly longer than the stride length of the control group.

Ulrich et al. (2008) extended the evaluation of the higher-intensity and lower-intensity intervention protocols started by Wu et al. (2007). The conditions available for the two protocols were matching those previously described by Wu et al. The authors wanted to determine the effects of the protocols on the children's frequencies of alternating steps and on the onset of a variety of locomotor skills (e.g., moving forward using prewalking methods and raising self to stand). Data showed that the frequencies of alternating steps were similar at the start of the study, favored the children with lower-intensity protocol during the earlier parts of the intervention and the children with higher-intensity protocol during the later parts of the intervention. The attainment of all basic locomotor milestones occurred at an earlier age for the children with higher-intensity protocol. However, differences between groups were statistically significant only on moving forward using prewalking methods and rising to a standing position.

Angulo-Barroso et al. (2008a, b) and Wu et al. (2008) compared the effects of the different treadmill intervention conditions (i.e., higher- and lower-intensity protocols) on longer-term performance of the children experiencing the intervention. Angulo-Barroso et al. (2008a) examined the level (intensity) of physical activity of the children who had followed the higher- and lower-intensity treadmill protocols for 1 year after the end of the intervention protocols. For that purpose, they analyzed the children's engagement data in terms of sedentary-to-light activity and moderate-to-vigorous activity and differentiated the activity in trunk and legs activity. The results suggested that children who had experienced the higher-intensity treadmill protocol continued to have a higher level (longer periods) of intense activity during the follow-up year. This finding was considered particularly relevant in view of the fact that children with Down syndrome tend to be less active and less energetic/intense than their typical counterparts.

Angulo-Barroso et al. (2008b) conducted a 1-year follow-up study to determine the long-term effects of higher- and lower-intensity treadmill protocols on children's gait. Six gait parameters were examined: step length, step width, normalized velocity, cadence, double support percentage, and dynamic base. Data showed that both groups of children had a significant increase in normalized velocity, cadence, step length, and dynamic base and a decrease of step width and double support percentage over the follow-up. The children experiencing the higher-intensity protocol produced significantly higher normalized velocity and cadence and lower double support percentages compared to the children with lower-intensity protocol.

Wu et al. (2008) collected 1-year follow-up data on obstacle clearance for the children who had experienced higher- and lower-intensity treadmill protocols until they reached walking criterion. The follow-up data collection concerned the way the children approached and cleared obstacles that they encountered on the walking pattern. The height of the obstacles increased over the various assessments carried out through the follow-up period. Overall findings showed that all children increased the percentages of walking (and reduced percentages of crawling) over the obstacle. Yet the percentages of walking of the children who had experienced a higher-intensity treadmill protocol were significantly larger than those of the children who had experienced the lower-intensity protocol. This difference suggested that the first group of children had managed a greater development in adaptive gait.

Looper and Ulrich (2010) extended the research scope of the previous studies by assessing the possible influence of early orthosis use with treadmill intervention. At the start of the study, 12 children were allocated to the control group receiving treadmill intervention, and 10 children were allocated to the experimental group receiving treadmill intervention and orthosis use. The study started when the children could pull themselves to a standing position and continued until they had 1 month of independent walking experience. Treadmill intervention stopped 1 month earlier (i.e., at the onset of independent walking). Treadmill intervention was introduced in small steps (i.e., using 1-min walking followed by 1-min rest) before being carried out in an uninterrupted session. The length of the intervention sessions was planned to be 8 min (even though parents seemed to eventually manage sessions of about 6 min). Sessions were carried out 5 days a week. Children of the experimental group were also to wear a supramalleolar orthosis for several hours a day. The children's progress was evaluated through the overall scores on the gross motor function measure (GMFM; Russell et al. 2002), as well as through the scores on the specific domains of this measure, that is, crawling and kneeling, standing, and walking, running, and jumping. All the children showed large improvements in their overall scores on the GMFM as well as on the single domains (scales) of this measure over time. The scores at 1 month after walking onset (i.e., at the end of the study) showed that the control group scored significantly higher than the experimental group on the GMFM total score, the standing scale score, and the walking, running, and jumping scale score.

Participants with Cerebral Palsy and Rett Syndrome

The studies carried out with these participants resorted to the use of partial body weight support to help the participants respond appropriately and avoid rapid tiredness. Schindl et al. (2000) carried out a study with ten participants with cerebral palsy (and possible intellectual and communicative disabilities), whose ages ranged from 6 to 18 years with a mean of over 11 years. Six of these participants, who presented with tetraparesis, were not able to walk at all unless firm support was provided to them. Of the remaining four participants, two required support for balance and/or coordination, one needed verbal supervision and occasional physical support, and one could walk in an athetoid manner. The participants received different levels of body weight support in line with what was required by their general situation. Two therapists would be available at the sides of the treadmill to facilitate their step movements and their leg and foot positions and also to ensure that they would not sit on the harness supporting them. The treadmill was set at speeds ranging from 0.14 to 0.42 m/s at the beginning of the intervention. The speeds were gradually increased and reached ranges of 0.25–0.47 m/s by the end of the study. The net walking ranged from about 10 to 19 min at the beginning of the study and increased gradually for eight of the participants while remained virtually the same for two of them (i.e., two participants who showed signs of fatigue). The program lasted 3 months and involved three 30-min sessions a week. Participants were encouraged to walk continuously for periods of 5–10 min followed by rest periods. Prior to the start of the study, all participants had been familiarizing with treadmill sessions. Group results showed significant improvements in standing and walking. Of the six participants of the first group (i.e., those with more severe neuromotor impairment), five were reported to have an improvement of their standing and walking abilities. All four participants of the second group showed improvement in standing (and postural abilities) and in walking.

Dodd and Foley (2007) sought to determine whether a 6-week program involving treadmill sessions with partial body weight support could increase (a) the self-selected, overground walking speed and (b) the walking endurance of participants with cerebral palsy and intellectual/developmental disabilities. To answer those questions, the authors compared the performance of seven participants who were provided with 12 treadmill sessions of up to 30 min with the performance of seven matched, control participants. The participants were reportedly walking with different levels of supports and were 5.4–14.6 ($M=8.9$) years old. Partial body weight support and treadmill speed were adjusted through the sessions provided to the experimental group. Results showed that this group had a significant increase in self-selected overground speed as indicated by the 10-m walking test. Indeed, six of the seven members of the group showed an improvement on their selected speed at the test, compared to their baseline performance on it. By contrast, only two members of the control group showed an improvement in their speed. Some improvement also occurred in their overground walking endurance as indicated by the 10-min walking test. Five members of the experimental (vs. three of the control group) had an improvement on this test.

Borggraefe et al. (2008) carried out a study with a 6-year-old child who was diagnosed with bilateral spastic cerebral palsy and some level of intellectual and adaptive disability. The child was able to walk with an assistive mobility device and was able to communicate possible pain and discomfort. The aim was to assess the impact of 12 treadmill sessions carried out over a period of 3 weeks. The sessions lasted over 30 min during which the child was shown preferred videos to motivate his participation. Initially, about 50 % of the child's body weight was supported during the sessions. Such support decreased to nearly zero by the end of the intervention. The treadmill speed was set at 0.27 m/s at the start of the study and increased across sessions. The child showed marked improvement in overground walking velocity on the 10-m walking test (i.e., from about 0.25 to about 0.60 m/s), and his speed was preserved at a 4-month follow-up. Similarly positive data were obtained on the 6-min walking test (i.e., from a distance of 55 m to a distance of 115 m, which became 152 at the 6-month follow-up). GMFM scores also improved with regard to the standing domain as well as on the walking, running, and jumping domains (Russell et al. 2002).

Willoughby et al. (2010) (a) assessed the safety and feasibility of a treadmill intervention program with partial body weight support within a special school environment and (b) compared the effects of the aforementioned program with those of overground walking practice on the walking endurance, walking speed, and walking function of participants with cerebral palsy and moderate to severe intellectual disability. Twenty-six participants of 5–18 years of age (mean of about 11 years) were included in the study: 12 were involved in the treadmill intervention program and 14 in the overground walking practice. The treadmill program involved two sessions per week for 9 weeks. The body weight support was systematically reduced in relation to the participants' improvement. The treadmill speed was gradually increased to levels tolerable for the participants. Participants were helped with standing upright and performing the gait cycle. A mirror was also available as a way to provide them feedback as to the postural condition and promote motivation. The overground (control) program involved the use of a walking/supporting device through which the participants could practice walking in the school corridors or on the grounds. The staff could provide assistance with the components of the gait cycle. At each session, the participants were encouraged to walk faster and for a longer duration. The maximum walking time across conditions was 30 min. Sessions could be interrupted if the participants asked to do so or stopped walking. There were no significant differences between the two programs in terms of their overall effects (i.e., walking speed, walking endurance, and walking function). Also, none of the participants suffered any adverse events or negative safety issues during the treadmill intervention program or the control program. Thus, both programs can be considered safe and feasible within school contexts.

Lotan et al. (2004b) conducted a study with four girls with Rett syndrome whose ages were between 8.5 and 11 years (with a mean of 10 years). The girls were provided with treadmill intervention over a period of 2 months, during which they had 36–50 treadmill sessions. Initially, the sessions lasted 5 min. Then they were gradually increased to a maximum of 30 min. Eventually, their length was set at about 20 min. The maximum speed of the treadmill was about 0.42 m/s, and the inclination remained at the zero level. During the sessions, the girls were presented with their preferred songs and music. Functional effects of the treadmill intervention were measured through a multi-item motor functioning scale set up for the study. The items on which the authors found significant differences/improvements between pre- and postintervention measurements were those concerning (a) knee walking, (b) walking speed over a 25-m distance, (c) speed in descending a staircase of three stairs, and (d) speed in ascending the same staircase.

Table 6.2 Studies using walkers with microswitches and contingent stimulation

Studies	Participants	Age (years)	Microswitches
Lancioni et al. (2004)	1	19	Two optic microswitches at the heels
Lancioni et al. (2005a)	1	13	Two optic microswitches (one on the walker's side and one on a shoe)
Lancioni et al. (2005b)	2	11, 47	Two optic microswitches on the walker's sides
Lancioni et al. (2007a)	4	7–41	Two optic microswitches at the heels or one optic microswitch on the side of a leg
Lancioni et al. (2007b)	2	8, 10	Two pressure microswitches under the shoes or two optic microswitches at the heels
Lancioni et al. (2008)	2	3, 12	Two optic microswitches on the walker's sides
Lancioni et al. (2010)	5	5.5–11	Two optic microswitches on the walker's sides, or two pressure microswitches under the shoes, or one pressure microswitch under a shoe

Studies Reporting the Combined Use of Walker Devices and Microswitches

In these studies, the walker devices ensured the participants' upright posture and could also provide them partial body weight support (through a saddle or harness) so as to facilitate their performance of step responses (or of other foot-leg movements). The microswitches monitored the occurrence of the target responses and allowed them to be followed by an automatic (contingent) delivery of brief periods of preferred stimulation. This aspect was considered of critical importance to motivate the participants to make an effort to take independent steps and have a positive (happy) experience of the sessions (Green and Reid 1999a, b; Lancioni et al. 2005b, c; Miltenberger 2004). Seven studies (see Table 6.2) reported the use of walker devices and microswitches with contingent stimulation for participants with multiple disabilities, that is, intellectual, motor and, often, also sensory disabilities. Their level of intellectual disability was rated in the severe to profound range. Six studies were aimed at promoting stepping responses (locomotion) with a total of 15 participants (Lancioni et al. 2004, 2005a, b, 2007a, 2008, 2010). The seventh study targeted preambulatory leg-foot movements of two children (Lancioni et al. 2007b).

Lancioni et al. (2005a), for example, worked with an adolescent of 13 years of age who was rated in the profound intellectual disability range, was totally blind, and presented with spastic tetraparesis and scoliosis. He could stand and briefly walk only if he received extensive physical support from a person or used a four-wheel support walker. His performance with the walker was, however, reported to be fairly modest with only a low frequency of steps taken. This was thought to be largely due to a motivation problem (i.e., disinterest in making an effort without positive/reinforcing consequences for it). To increase his motivation to walk, two optic microswitches with contingent stimulation were used in combination with the walker. One microswitch was attached to the right lateral panel of the walker to monitor the steps the participant made with his right foot. The other microswitch was attached to his left shoe to detect steps he made with his left foot. The microswitches were connected to an electronic control system, which was attached to the walker frame. Microswitch activation triggered the control system, which in turn, activated recording devices (available with the control system), which played preferred music or recorded praise statements. The study was carried out according to an ABAB sequence in which A represented baseline phases and B intervention phases. Baseline and intervention phases involved two to four 5-min sessions per day. During intervention sessions, the occurrence of a step (the activation of one of the microswitches) caused the occurrence of 3 s of preferred stimulation. During the first baseline, the participant's mean frequency of steps per session was about 45. During the first intervention phase, the mean frequency increased to over 100 per session. During the second baseline, the frequency declined. During the second intervention, it increased again above 100. Data also showed that during the intervention phases, the participant had an increase in indices of happiness (i.e., smiles or excited vocalizations).

Lancioni et al. (2005b) worked with a child and a woman of 11 and 47 years of age, respectively. Both participants were rated in the profound intellectual disability range. They presented with spastic tetraparesis and scoliosis, could only walk with support, and were familiar with the use of a four-wheel support walker. The walker was fitted with a saddle, a feet divider, and a frame passing under the participants' arms and around their chest. As with the previous case, these participants' frequencies of steps while on the walker were relatively modest, and thus, microswitches and contingent stimulation were included in the intervention program. The microswitches (i.e., optic sensors) were (a) attached to the left and right panels of the walker device, respectively, so that they could detect steps performed with the left and the right foot and (b) connected to an electronic control system, which regulated the occurrence of preferred stimulation. The intervention was carried out after baseline phases of different lengths for the two participants (i.e., according to a multiple baseline design across participants) and involved three or four 5-min sessions per day. The performance of steps led to 3 s of preferred stimulation. Data showed that the participants had mean frequencies of 24 and 70 steps per session during the baseline and 103 and 194 steps per session during the intervention. The participants also showed increases of indices of happiness indicating that they enjoyed their walking performance.

Lancioni et al. (2007a) used the aforementioned approach with two children of about 7 and 9 years of age, and a man and a woman of 19 and 41 years of age. One of the children presented with spastic tetraparesis and visual impairment; the other child had low muscle tone and visual and auditory impairments. Both adults presented with spastic tetraparesis. One of them also had severe visual impairment. All participants were considered to function in the profound intellectual disability range but could stand and take some steps with support. They were provided with four-wheel support walkers, which for three of them also included a harness securing them and lifting part of their weight. The walkers were combined with microswitches, control systems, and, during the intervention, with contingent stimulation as well. Microswitches varied across participants. For two of them, optic microswitches were attached to the heels of their shoes. For the other two, only one microswitch was used, and this was attached to the external side of the right leg, slightly above the ankle. During intervention, the control system ensured (a) the occurrence of 2.5 s of preferred stimulation at each step (for the former two participants) and (b) the occurrence of 5 or 6 s of preferred stimulation at each microswitch activation (for the latter two participants). Participants usually received several 5-min sessions per day according to an ABAB sequence in which A represented periods of baseline sessions (with no stimulation) and B represented periods of intervention sessions (with contingent stimulation). The results showed that all participants (a) had relatively low frequencies of step responses during the first baseline, (b) increased those frequencies greatly during the first intervention phase, (c) showed drastic frequency declines during the second baseline, and (d) restored high frequencies during the second intervention phase. All participants also showed increases in indices of happiness, such as smiles, during the intervention phases.

Lancioni et al. (2010) extended the approach to five new children between about 5.5 and 11 years of age. They were reported to be in the severe or profound intellectual disability ranges and presented with spastic tetraparesis. Four of them also showed different levels of visual impairment. All children could walk with extensive physical support from a caregiver or through the use of four-wheel walkers equipped with a frame passing around their chest and under their arms and a harness or saddle securing their posture and lifting part of their body weight. Yet their frequency of steps (i.e., their motivation to walk) seemed quite modest, so the use of microswitches and contingent stimulation (i.e., preferred stimulation following the performance of steps) was added as in the studies reviewed above. The position and characteristics of the microswitches varied across participants in an attempt to increase their efficiency and practicality. For two of the participants, the microswitches were fixed to the right and left panels of the walker device so that they could monitor step responses with the right and left foot. For two other participants, the microswitches were attached to the shoes. For the fifth participant, only one microswitch was used, and it was connected to his left foot. The study was carried out according to an ABAB sequence (see above) for four of the five participants and a simple AB for the fifth participant and involved several 5-min sessions per day. During the intervention (B) phases, steps were followed by brief periods of preferred stimulation. The stimulation varied from 3 to 5 s for the four participants who used two microswitches and lasted 8 s for the fifth participant who used only one microswitch. During the initial baseline, the participant' mean frequencies of steps varied between 7 and 26 per session. During the first intervention phase, the mean frequencies varied between 23 and 110 per session. The frequencies declined during the second baseline and increased again during the second intervention phase (i.e., for the four participants with the ABAB sequence).

Lancioni et al. (2007b) used the same approach to foster preambulatory foot-leg movements of two children of 8 and 10 years of age. The study involved an ABAB sequence and adopted technological and procedural conditions similar to those of the studies summarized above. The difference from the other studies concerned the responses targeted. These were not regular steps but foot-leg movements preliminary to them, that is, foot-leg movements that ended with the child's foot touching the floor (after any minimal lifting from it), in a way that resembled a side, forward, or backward step. These movements were followed by 5 s of preferred stimulation during the intervention phases of the study. Baseline and intervention phases were carried out through 5-min sessions repeated three to five times during the day. Both children started with relatively low baseline levels (i.e., 18 and 14 movements per session) and increased those levels drastically during the first intervention (i.e., reached mean frequencies of 52 and 82 movements per session). The second baseline led to a drop of responding. The second intervention phase increased the mean frequencies to 58 and 129 movements for the two participants, respectively.

Discussion

Outcome of the Studies Using a Robot

The studies included in the overview concerned three different forms of assistive technology (i.e., robot, treadmills, and walkers combined with microswitches and contingent stimulation), which seemed adequate to promote relevant outcomes emphasizing different educational and rehabilitation target areas. The studies using the robot were not really aimed at enhancing walking skills or establishing new levels of walking performance as such but rather at ensuring a technology-supported walking behavior that was instrumental for the participants' activity engagement and physical exercise (Lancioni et al. 1993b, 2000a). Indeed, the robot seemed to work in a satisfactory manner to promote the participants' independence from the staff, increase their engagement opportunities, and extend their overall walking time and distance (i.e., allowing walking to become a basic opportunity of mild physical exercise; Lancioni et al. 2000a).

The robot's effectiveness was clearly connected to the fact that the participants were capable of walking with support and required only a steady object to use for that purpose. The robot's role, however, was not only that of being a steady object and supporting the participants during their walking but also that of leading/guiding them through the space that they had to travel to reach the target destinations. This second aspect was critical given the fact that the participants presented with visual impairment or blindness and had most serious orientation problems (see Chap. 5).

The activities carried out by the participants at the destinations that they reached with the robot differed in relation to their basic characteristics and abilities. More skillful participants were provided with the opportunity to choose and perform constructive, vocational activities (Lancioni et al. 1993b). Less skillful participants were only required to perform simple object transportation and object disposal (setting away), but the staff considered this engagement together with the independent walking socially/practically relevant and desirable (Lancioni et al. 1994, 1997).

Further analysis and generalization of the aforementioned results would require some caution due to two methodological/research limitations of the studies reviewed. The first limitation concerns the fact that the number of persons involved in the studies was small (i.e., a total of seven participants) (Kazdin 2001; Richards et al. 1999). The second limitation concerns the fact that all the studies were carried out by the same research unit, within a single rehabilitation and care cultural context (Lancioni et al. 1993b, 1994, 1997, 2000a).

Outcome of the Studies Using Treadmills

The use of the treadmill with children with Down syndrome seemed to promote earlier achievement of basic milestones, such as rising to stand, walking with help, and walking independently (Ulrich et al. 2001). Higher-intensity-individualized intervention (involving a rise in demands tailored to individual progress) seemed more effective than a lower-intensity-generalized intervention protocol (Wu et al. 2007). However, the differences between the two protocols reached levels of statistical significance only on moving forward using prewalking methods and rising to a standing position (Ulrich et al. 2008). Higher-intensity-individualized intervention seemed also to have positive, long-term effects, that is, it was associated with (a) higher levels and longer duration of intense activity, (b) higher normalized velocity and cadence and lower double support percentages, and (c) higher percentages of walking (and reduced percentages of crawling) over obstacles (Angulo-Barroso et al. 2008a, b; Lloyd et al. 2010; Wu et al. 2008). The addition of a supramalleolar orthosis to treadmill intervention did not seem to bring about improvements in the outcome. To the contrary, children of the control group scored significantly higher than the experimental group on the GMFM total score, the standing scale score, and the walking, running, and jumping scale score.

These findings seem convincing in suggesting that the treadmill intervention and, in particular, the higher-intensity-individualized protocol can have beneficial effects in promoting the achievement of independent walking and other locomotor skills relevant for development and adaptive performance. The questions one can raise are whether (a) the treadmill continues to be the only exercise/practice means after the initial period or other overground forms of technology (e.g., walkers and microswitches) may also be used and (b) the parents/caregivers' approval, encouragement, and praise are sufficiently reinforcing events for the treadmill exercise or other sensory events could also be programmed to increase the child's motivation to perform (Kazdin 2001; Lancioni et al. 2010; Vashdi et al. 2008).

The use of the treadmill with persons with cerebral palsy indicated that participants of different levels of disability had an improvement of their standing and walking abilities after relatively brief intervention periods. Marked improvement was found in overground walking velocity on the 10-m walking test and in walking endurance on the 6-min walking test (Borggraefe et al. 2008; Dodd and Foley 2007). Yet the effects of treadmill intervention did not seem to differ significantly from the effects of a control program involving the use of a walking/supporting device through which the participants could practice walking in the school corridors (i.e., overground) (Willoughby et al. 2010). This particular finding seems to cast some doubts as to the specificity of the treadmill intervention per se and to emphasize instead an intervention approach that involves increased walking practice and exercise regardless of the means through which these specific objectives are pursued and realized (Begnoche et al. 2005; Hayakawa and Kobayashi 2011).

A second point that was raised above and applies again here is that of motivation. Of the four studies directed at participants with cerebral palsy, only two seemed to consider this issue. One was explicit about using reinforcing events (preferred videos and movies) during treadmill walking (Borggraefe et al. 2008), while the other used a mirror as a source of feedback and possible motivation (Willoughby et al. 2010). The limited emphasis on motivation and reinforcement could represent a clear weakness of these intervention programs. In fact, they require the participants to produce a large effort on the basis of a goal that might be too far and too difficult for them to appreciate (i.e., insufficiently motivating) given their disabilities. A recent study by Vashdi et al. (2008) was aimed at providing some clarification on this issue. The authors compared four different conditions that were activated during the treadmill walking of a group of 13 children ranging in age from 5.5 to 11 years. The conditions consisted of a close proximity of the supervisor, a distant presence of the supervisor, the use of positive reinforcement (i.e., the use of videos with movies), and paired modeling (the use of two treadmills with two children involved in the walking in parallel). The dependent variable was the participants' attempts to discontinue their walking during the sessions. The results of the study showed that the use of the reinforcement led (a) to a significantly smaller number of attempts to discontinue walking than the close proximity and distant presence of the supervisor but (b) to a significantly larger number of attempts than paired modeling. The authors argued that the positive reinforcement condition may have failed to be the strongest (most effective) condition simply because it presented weaknesses in terms of the stimuli included (i.e., not selected for the individual children) and in terms of its application (i.e., at fixed intervals).

The use of the treadmill for children with Rett syndrome led to a generally positive outcome in knee walking, walking speed over a 25-m distance, and speed in descending and ascending a staircase of three stairs. These results, although encouraging, may need to be taken with great caution given the fact that they are based on only one study with four participants (Lotan et al. 2004b). An interesting (positive) aspect of the intervention program was that it included the use of positive reinforcement stimuli (preferred songs and music) to motivate the participants to engage in treadmill walking.

Outcome of the Studies Using Walkers and Microswitches

The studies using walkers with microswitches and preferred stimulation contingent on the participants' steps (or foot-leg movements) presented consistently positive results in terms of steps/movements' increases. This favorable outcome may, first of all, be ascribed to the fact that the participants selected for inclusion were largely suitable to the programs. That is, they possessed (i.e., except those included in the study on foot-leg movements) the basic stepping skills required for progressing toward satisfactory supported ambulation. Secondly, the use of preferred stimulation contingent on the step responses appeared to be motivating (reinforcing) and therefore succeeded in strengthening the participants' efforts to walk and in increasing their overall frequencies of steps.

The finding that the increase in the frequencies of step responses was accompanied by increases in indices of happiness seems to make the program package more interesting and respectful of the participants and of their quality of life (Lancioni et al. 2005a, b, 2007a). Indeed, the increase in indices of happiness may be taken to suggest that the stimulation provided largely exceeded the efforts required by the walking performance and the participants were able to enjoy the experience (Dillon and Carr 2007; Green and Reid 1999a, b; Green et al. 2005; Horton and Taylor 1989; Lalli et al. 1994; Lancioni et al. 2005c; Strawbridge et al. 1989).

Although no specific measurements were taken as to the technical aspects of walking per se, one would reasonably expect the general walking performance to improve as a consequence of the extended practice the participants experienced with regular daily recurrence (Anttila et al. 2008; Blundell et al. 2003; Day et al. 2004; Hamed and Abd-elwahab 2011; Ketelaar et al. 2001; Kollen 2009).

Questions may be raised as to whether the participants of the Lancioni et al.'s (2007b) study (i.e., those exposed to the program in which simple foot-leg movements were followed by preferred stimulation) could have benefited more from a treadmill intervention protocol. Indeed, a treadmill intervention would have made the participants exercise the step cycle and the muscle components involved in the performance of it. By contrast, the program carried out in the study reported did not target the step cycle but rather focused on the participants' initiative and motivation to carry out basic movements that could develop into functional step/travel instruments (Borggraefe et al. 2008; Willoughby et al. 2010).

Implications of the Studies' Outcomes

The results obtained with the use of the different approaches and the comments provided about them may have important implications on two specific grounds. On the one hand, they seem to provide a set of data that constitutes an encouraging basis in favor of direct (functional) intervention for promoting ambulatory behavior and against the need of relying exclusively (predominantly) on the neurodevelopmental method (Begnoche and Pitetti 2007; Day et al. 2004; Ketelaar et al. 2001). On the other hand, they provide a variety of specific examples (and relevant observations) that can be viewed as forms of practical intervention guidance for regular rehabilitation settings as well as home/family contexts (Bodkin et al. 2003; Palisano et al. 2003; Zwicker and Mayson 2010; Tieman et al. 2004; Wu et al. 2007). For example, the use of the treadmill, which might be considered a plausible strategy for many persons with cerebral palsy and multiple disabilities, may need to be programmed in combination with positive stimulation. This stimulation would be critical to motivate the person to endure the effort required by the situation (and thus avoid attempts to discontinue the walking engagement or to show other problem behaviors) and improve the overall mood and possibly display indices of happiness (Vashdi et al. 2008). Obviously, the stimulation is to be selected for the single persons specifically to maximize its positive impact on their behavior (Kazdin 2001; Lancioni et al. 2010; Vashdi et al. 2008).

The use of treadmills and the use of walkers with microswitches and contingent stimulation, which have been reported as two different approaches directed at persons with possibly different characteristics, might not need to be viewed as completely separate. In fact, one might argue that the two approaches can represent two segments of the same rehabilitation program for many persons (Lancioni et al. 2010; Willoughby et al. 2010). For example, the first segment could involve the use of the treadmill to help staff or parents establish basic stepping responses and eventually promote walking performance with partial levels of body weight support. The second segment could involve the use of the walker and microswitches, which would provide posture control and body weight support and ensure the presence of contingent stimulation to guarantee a successful practice of the new skills (Ketelaar et al. 2001; Lancioni et al. 2007a, 2009b).

Once the person has acquired the ability to walk with some form of support, he or she should probably be enabled to use such a new skill as a means to reach target places and carry out specific activities. In this way, the new walking skill would be fully integrated within the person's education/rehabilitation plan. The use of the walker device with microswitches would be the best solution to ensure the achievement of this goal for its flexibility in allowing different travel routes, for its possibility of providing stimulation contingent on walking, as well as for its practicality and affordability (see below).

The question of whether the provision of stimulation for the step responses would remain necessary cannot be answered in general. One might hypothesize that most persons with severe/profound and multiple disabilities and extensive neuromotor impairment (a) would continue to find walking a demanding task rather than a simple and enjoyable engagement, (b) would not have particular interests in exploring the environment and reaching specific places (i.e., may not possess specific/intrinsic motivation for walking as such), and (c) would not find self-fulfillment and satisfaction in performing most of the daily activities available for them to perform. For these persons, the question then might be not whether to eliminate the stimulation for the step responses but rather when and how to reduce this stimulation from a continuous basis to an intermittent level (Lancioni et al. 2005a, b, 2010). A different perspective may exist for persons who have a less serious disability situation. They could find the walking engagement less demanding, and their walking and activity performance could be maintained through the reinforcing events that normally follow the completion of the activities (Kazdin 2001; Lancioni et al. 2000a, 2005b, 2007a).

Practical Considerations on the Use of the Different Technologies

The different technologies can easily be viewed as complementary tools in a complex intervention job such as that directed at establishing some level of walking and integrating it (making it functional) within the education/rehabilitation program designed for the person (Begnoche and Pitetti 2007; Kollen et al. 2009; Lancioni et al. 2009b; Simard-Tremblay et al. 2010). The treadmill is the basic technology, that is, the only resource one can use at the beginning of the process when the person does not have walking skills. At this preliminary level, the treadmill can also be combined with an assistive mobility device that helps the therapist in ensuring the person's performance of the step cycle (Borggraefe et al. 2008). Obviously, the combined use of the two would complicate the procedure, require higher levels of professional expertise, and limit the application of the intervention sessions to specialized places rather than conventional daily contexts (Damiano and DeJong 2009; Lancioni et al. 2009b). In practice, the availability of these resources and the expertise to apply them properly may not be widely expected.

The treadmill may remain a basic exercise instrument that maintains (or enhances) the person's skills long after the person has acquired the initial walking levels (Zwicker and Mayson 2010). Two clarifications need, however, to be made at this point. First, the use of the treadmill may require to be reconsidered with the view of ensuring the person's motivation to exercise walking through the delivery of positive (reinforcing) stimulation. Second, the treadmill cannot be seen as a tool to help persons who walk with support to practice their skill level functionally within their daily context. In fact, these persons would be expected to make their walking part of their occupational engagement and manage to reach different activity destinations, with beneficial consequences for their adaptive behavior and their social status (Lancioni et al. 2009b; Maher et al. 2011; Whittingham et al. 2010; Van Gestel et al. 2008).

The only way these persons can integrate walking with daily activities is through the use of the robot or the walker with microswitches. The robot has the advantage of guiding the persons to the destinations and avoiding any orientation problems. The fact that it does not provide stimulation for the step responses could be overcome by adding a stimulation source that becomes active in connection with the robot's movement (Lancioni et al. 2000b, 2008). This combination could make its use not only effective but also relatively pleasant for the person thus preventing (minimizing) problem behaviors (e.g., Vashdi et al. 2008) and possibly increasing indices of happiness (Dillon and Carr 2007; Green and Reid 1999a, b; Green et al.

2005; Lancioni et al. 2005a, b, c, 2007a). The real problem with the robot is that it cannot be considered a practical and affordable technology for families and daily contexts. These specific reasons largely explain why the early studies were not followed by new research initiatives directed at developing further (upgraded) versions of the robot and at assessing new applications of it for promoting ambulation and activity (Claxton et al. 2011; Hubbard Winkler et al. 2010; Lancioni et al. 2001, 2005b, 2008).

The use of walkers with microswitches and contingent stimulation may be viewed as the only real option to promote the integration of supported walking into the daily occupational program of the person. Indeed, walkers are widely available and can be supplemented with microswitches and stimulus sources for a relatively accessible cost. In this way, they become the technology that staff and parents can resort to in the longer term and for most part of the day. The question of whether stimulation should be maintained on a consistent basis has been addressed above. For some (most difficult) cases, it would be expected to remain indispensable, and thus, it would need to occur consistently. For other (less difficult) cases, the stimulation may be reduced into some form of intermittent scheme (Kazdin 2001; Miltenberger 2004). In both situations, the ultimate goals would be to preserve the participant's motivation to walk and to ensure the participant's satisfaction (happiness) through the walking time (Lancioni et al. 2007a; Samuelsson and Wressle 2008). In order to achieve these goals, the stimulation available would need to be reviewed regularly and adapted to the participants' preferences.

Conclusions

The studies reviewed and the following discussion seem to underline among others that (a) the three approaches (the three forms of technology) were met with encouraging results; (b) caution is needed in interpreting the results obtained with the use of the robot due to the fairly small number of participants involved, in addition to the fact that the studies were carried out by the same research group; (c) the use of the treadmill and the use of the walker with microswitches (or of the robot) may be seen as two segments of the same rehabilitation program for a large number of persons; (d) the notion of walking motivation needs to be tackled within treadmill-based programs to avoid problem behavior and promote positive mood; and (e) the use of the robot, although apparently promising in terms of impact, may not be considered a really plausible option in practice due to the cost problems (Dillon and Carr 2007; Kazdin 2001; Lancioni et al. 2001; Samuelsson and Wressle 2008; Vashdi et al. 2008).

Any new developments in this area may require specific research efforts. One such effort could be directed at assessing (a) ways of arranging positive stimulation within treadmill-based intervention programs, (b) possible benefits of such stimulation in terms of participants' general behavioral compliance and mood (indices of happiness), and (c) social validation ratings of treadmill-based intervention situations with and without positive stimulation (cf. Green and Reid 1999a, b; Lalli et al. 1994; Lancioni et al. 2005c). The social validation assessment could involve the employment of family members, rehabilitation personnel, as well as service organizers in the position of raters (Callahan et al. 2008; Lancioni et al. 2006; Storey 1996).

A second research effort could investigate ways of coordinating treadmill-based programs and programs based on the use of walkers with microswitches and contingent stimulation within practical rehabilitation situations. For example, participants could be initially exposed to the treadmill program (i.e., to a higher-intensity version of it with the addition of positive stimulation) to develop basic stepping (walking) responses. Subsequently, they could be shifted to the use of a walker with microswitches and contingent stimulation to foster self-determination and integrate walking with daily activities (Ketelaar et al. 2001; Lancioni et al. 2009b; Palisano et al. 2003).

A third research effort could be directed to determining whether it is possible to develop a new form of technology which is simpler and more affordable than the robot previously used but allows the participants to receive prompts for walking and direction cues so as to promote the walking performance and facilitate the orientation to the activity destinations (Borg et al. 2011; Brown et al. 2009; Deutsch 2009; Green 2010).

References

Accivatti, C., Harro, C. C., & Bothner, K. E. (2006). The effect of body weight supported treadmill training on gait function in children with cerebral palsy. *Pediatric Physical Therapy, 18*, 82–83.

Angulo-Barroso, R., Burghardt, A. R., Lloyd, M., & Ulrich, D. A. (2008a). Physical activity in infants with Down syndrome receiving a treadmill intervention. *Infant Behavior & Development, 31*, 255–269.

Angulo-Barroso, R. M., Wu, J., & Ulrich, D. A. (2008b). Long-term effect of different treadmill interventions on gait development in new walkers with Down syndrome. *Gait & Posture, 27*, 231–238.

Anttila, H., Autti-Rämö, I., Suoranta, J., Mäkelä, M., & Malmivaara, A. (2008). Effectiveness of physical therapy interventions for children with cerebral palsy: A systematic review. *BMC Pediatrics, 8*, 14.

Bar-Haim, S., Harries, N., Belokopytov, M., Frank, A., Copeliovitch, L., Kaplanski, J., & Lahat, E. (2006). A comparison of efficacy of Adeli suit and neurodevelopmental treatments in children with cerebral palsy. *Developmental Medicine and Child Neurology, 48*, 325–330.

Beard, L. M., Harro, C., & Bothner, K. E. (2005). The effect of body weight support treadmill training on gait function in cerebral palsy: Two case studies. *Pediatric Physical Therapy, 17*, 72.

Begnoche, D., & Pitetti, K. H. (2007). Effects of traditional treatment and partial body weight treadmill training on the motor skills of children with spastic cerebral palsy: A pilot study. *Pediatric Physical Therapy, 19*, 11–19.

Begnoche, D., Sanders, E., & Pitetti, K. H. (2005). Effect of an intensive physical therapy program with partial body weight treadmill training on a 2 year-old child with spastic quadriplegic cerebral palsy. *Pediatric Physical Therapy, 17*, 73.

Blundell, S. W., Shepherd, R. B., Dean, C. M., Adams, R. D., & Cahill, B. M. (2003). Functional strength training in cerebral palsy: A pilot study of a group circuit training class for children aged 4–8 years. *Clinical Rehabilitation, 17*, 48–57.

Bobath, K. (1980). *A neurophysiological basis for the treatment of cerebral palsy* (Clinics in developmental medicine, Vol. 75). London: Spastic International Medical Publications.

Bobath, K., & Bobath, B. (1984). The neurodevelopmental treatment. In D. Scutton (Ed.), *Management of the motor disorders of children with cerebral palsy* (Clinics in developmental medicine, Vol. 90, pp. 6–18). London: Spastic International Medical Publications.

Bodkin, A. W., Baxter, R. S., & Heriza, C. B. (2003). Treadmill training for an infant born preterm with a grade III intraventricular hemorrhage. *Physical Therapy, 83*, 1107–1118.

Borg, J., Larson, S., & Ostegren, P. O. (2011). The right to assistive technology: For whom, for what, and by whom? *Disability and Society, 26*, 151–167.

Borggraefe, I., Meyer-Heim, A., Kumar, A., Schaefer, J. S., Berweck, S., & Heinen, F. (2008). Improved gait parameters after robotic-assisted locomotor treadmill therapy in a 6-year-old child with cerebral palsy. *Movement Disorders, 23*, 280–283.

Brown, R. I., Schalock, R. L., & Brown, I. (2009). Quality of life: Its application to persons with intellectual disabilities and their families – Introduction and overview. *Journal of Policy and Practice in Intellectual Disabilities, 6*, 2–6.

Callahan, K., Henson, R., & Cowan, A. K. (2008). Social validation of evidence-based practices in autism by parents, teachers, and administrators. *Journal of Autism and Developmental Disorders, 38*, 678–692.

Cernak, K., Stevens, V., Price, R., & Shumway-Cook, A. (2008). Locomotor training using body-weight support on a treadmill in conjunction with ongoing physical therapy in a child with severe cerebellar ataxia. *Physical Therapy, 88*, 88–97.

Cherng, R.-J., Liu, C.-F., Lau, T.-W., & Hong, R.-B. (2007). Effect of treadmill training with body weight support on gait and gross motor function in children with spastic cerebral palsy. *American Journal of Physical Medicine & Rehabilitation, 86*, 548–555.

Chia, L. C., Guelfi, K. J., & Licari, M. K. (2010). A comparison of the oxygen cost of locomotion in children with and without developmental coordination disorder. *Developmental Medicine and Child Neurology, 52*, 251–255.

Cirignano, S. M., Du, L., & Morgan, K. T. (2010). Promoting youth physical activity in the classroom through a comprehensive walking program. *Family and Consumer Sciences Research Journal, 39*, 161–172.

Claxton, K., Paulden, M., Gravelle, H., Brower, W., & Culyer, A. J. (2011). Discounting and decision making in the economic evaluation of health-care technologies. *Health Economics, 20*, 2–15.

Damiano, D. L., & DeJong, S. L. (2009). A systematic review of the effectiveness of treadmill training and body weight support in pediatric rehabilitation. *Journal of Neurologic Physical Therapy, 33*, 27–44.

Dannemiller, L., Heriza, P., Burtner, P., & Gutierrez, T. (2005). Partial weight bearing treadmill training in the home with young children with cerebral palsy: A study of feasibility and motor outcomes. *Pediatric Physical Therapy, 17*, 77–78.

Day, J. A., Fox, E. J., Lowe, J., Swales, H. B., & Behrman, A. L. (2004). Locomotor training with partial body weight support on a treadmill in a nonambulatory child with spastic tetraplegic cerebral palsy: A case report. *Pediatric Physical Therapy, 16*, 106–113.

DeJong, S. L., Stuberg, W. A., & Spady, K. L. (2005). Conditioning effects of partial body weight support treadmill training in children with cerebral palsy. *Pediatric Physical Therapy, 17*, 78.

Deutsch, J. E. (2009). Virtual reality and gaming systems to improve walking and mobility for musculoskeletal and neuromuscular conditions. *Studies in Health Technology and Informatics, 145*, 84–93.

Dillon, C. M., & Carr, J. E. (2007). Assessing indices of happiness and unhappiness in individuals with developmental disabilities: A review. *Behavioral Interventions, 22*, 229–244.

Dodd, K. J., & Foley, S. (2007). Partial body-weight-supported treadmill training can improve walking in children with cerebral palsy: A clinical controlled trial. *Developmental Medicine and Child Neurology, 49*, 101–105.

Green, C. (2010). Considering the value associated with innovation in health technology appraisal decisions (deliberations): A nice thing to do? *Applied Health Economics and Health Policy, 8*, 1–5.

Green, C. W., & Reid, D. H. (1999a). A behavioral approach to identifying sources of happiness and unhappiness among individuals with profound multiple disabilities. *Behavior Modification, 23*, 280–293.

Green, C. W., & Reid, D. H. (1999b). Reducing indices of unhappiness among individuals with profound multiple disabilities during therapeutic exercise routines. *Journal of Applied Behavior Analysis, 32*, 137–147.

Green, C. W., Reid, D. H., Rollyson, J. H., & Passante, S. C. (2005). An enriched teaching program for reducing resistance and indices of unhappiness among individuals with profound multiple disabilities. *Journal of Applied Behavior Analysis, 38*, 221–233.

Hamed, N. S., & Abd-elwahab, M. S. (2011). Pedometer-based gait training in children with spastic hemiparetic cerebral palsy: A randomized controlled study. *Clinical Rehabilitation, 25*, 157–165.

Hayakawa, K., & Kobayashi, K. (2011). Physical and motor skill training for children with intellectual disabilities. *Perceptual and Motor Skills, 112*, 573–580.

Horton, S. V., & Taylor, D. C. (1989). The use of behavior therapy and physical therapy to promote independent ambulation in a preschooler with mental retardation and cerebral palsy. *Research in Developmental Disabilities, 10*, 363–375.

Hubbard Winkler, S. L., Vogel, B., Hoenig, H., Cowper Ripley, D. C., Wu, S., Fitzgerald, S. G., Mann, W. C., & Reker, D. M. (2010). Cost, utilization, and policy of provision of assistive technology devices to veterans poststroke by Medicare and VA. *Medical Care, 48*, 558–562.

Katz-Leurer, M., Rotem, H., Keren, O., & Meyer, S. (2010). The immediate effect of treadmill walking on step variability in boys with a history of severe traumatic brain injury and typically developed controls. *Developmental Neurorehabilitation, 13*, 170–174.

Kazdin, A. E. (2001). *Behavior modification in applied settings* (6th ed.). New York: Wadsworth.

Ketelaar, M., Vermeer, A., Hart, H., Van Petegem-van Beek, E., & Helders, P. J. M. (2001). Effects of a functional therapy program on motor abilities of children with cerebral palsy. *Physical Therapy, 81*, 1534–1545.

Kollen, B. J., Lennon, S., Lyons, B., Wheatly-Smith, L., Scheper, M., Buurke, J. H., Halfens, J., Geurts, A. C. H., & Kwakkel, G. (2009). The effectiveness of the Bobath concept in stroke rehabilitation: What is the evidence? *Stroke, 40*, e89–e97.

Lalli, J. S., Mauk, J. E., Goh, H., & Merlino, J. (1994). Successful behavioral intervention to treat children who are reluctant to ambulate. *Developmental Medicine and Child Neurology, 36*, 625–629.

Lancioni, G. E., Bellini, D., Oliva, D., Guzzini, F., & Pirani, P. (1989). A robot for guiding multihandicapped blind persons to carry out familiar daily activities. *Journal of the Multihandicapped Person, 2*, 271–282.

Lancioni, G. E., Bellini, D., & Oliva, D. (1993a). A robot to provide multihandicapped blind persons with physical guidance and activity choices. *Journal of Developmental and Physical Disabilities, 5*, 337–348.

Lancioni, G. E., Bellini, D., & Oliva, D. (1993b). Building choice opportunities within a robot-assisted occupational program: A case study. *Behavioral Residential Treatment, 8*, 219–226.

Lancioni, G. E., Gigante, A., O'Reilly, M. F., & Oliva, D. (2000a). Evaluating mild physical exercise with two persons with profound multiple disabilities. *Journal of Visual Impairment and Blindness, 94*, 461–465.

Lancioni, G. E., Gigante, A., O'Reilly, M. F., Oliva, D., & Montironi, L. (2000b). Indoor travel and simple tasks as physical exercise for people with profound multiple disabilities. *Perceptual and Motor Skills, 91*, 211–216.

Lancioni, G. E., Oliva, D., & Signorino, M. (1994). Promoting ambulation and object manipulation in persons with multiple handicaps through the use of a robot. *Perceptual and Motor Skills, 79*, 843–848.

Lancioni, G. E., Oliva, D., & O'Reilly, M. F. (1997). Ambulation, object manipulation, and multiple disabilities: Extending the applicability of a robot. *Journal of Visual Impairment & Blindness, 91*, 53–60.

Lancioni, G. E., O'Reilly, M. F., & Basili, G. (2001). An overview of technological resources used in rehabilitation research with people with severe/profound and multiple disabilities. *Disability and Rehabilitation, 23*, 501–508.

Lancioni, G. E., Singh, N. N., O'Reilly, M. F., Oliva, D., Scalini, L., & Groeneweg, J. (2004). Improving assisted ambulation in a man with multiple disabilities through the use of a microswitch cluster. *Behavioural and Cognitive Psychotherapy, 32*, 245–249.

Lancioni, G. E., Singh, N. N., O'Reilly, M. F., Campodonico, F., Oliva, D., & Vigo, C. M. (2005a). Promoting walker-assisted step responses by an adolescent with multiple disabilities through automatically delivered stimulation. *Journal of Visual Impairment and Blindness, 99*, 109–113.

Lancioni, G. E., Singh, N. N., O'Reilly, M. F., Campodonico, F., Piazzolla, G., Scalini, L., & Oliva, D. (2005b). Impact of favorite stimuli automatically delivered on step responses of persons with multiple disabilities during their use of walker devices. *Research in Developmental Disabilities, 26*, 71–76.

Lancioni, G. E., Singh, N. N., O'Reilly, M. F., Oliva, D., & Basili, G. (2005c). An overview of research on increasing indices of happiness of people with severe/profound intellectual and multiple disabilities. *Disability and Rehabilitation, 27*, 83–93.

Lancioni, G. E., O'Reilly, M. F., Singh, N. N., Groeneweg, J., Bosco, A., Tota, A., Smaldone, A., Stasolla, F., Manfredi, F., Baccani, S., & Pidala, S. (2006). A social validation assessment of microswitch-based programs for persons with multiple disabilities employing teacher trainees and parents as raters. *Journal of Developmental and Physical Disabilities, 18*, 383–391.

Lancioni, G. E., Singh, N. N., O'Reilly, M. F., Sigafoos, J., Oliva, D., Piazzolla, G., Pidala, S., Smaldone, A., & Manfredi, F. (2007a). Automatically delivered stimulation for walker-assisted step responses: Measuring its effects in persons with multiple disabilities. *Journal of Developmental and Physical Disabilities, 19*, 1–13.

Lancioni, G. E., Singh, N. N., O'Reilly, M. F., Sigafoos, J., Oliva, D., Scalini, L., Castagnaro, F., & Di Bari, M. (2007b). Promoting foot-leg movements in children with multiple disabilities through the use of support devices and technology for regulating contingent stimulation. *Cognitive Processing, 8*, 279–283.

Lancioni, G. E., De Pace, C., Singh, N. N., O'Reilly, M. F., Sigafoos, J., & Didden, R. (2008). Promoting step responses of children with multiple disabilities through a walker device and microswitches with contingent stimuli. *Perceptual and Motor Skills, 107*, 114–118.

Lancioni, G. E., O'Reilly, M. F., Singh, N. N., Sigafoos, J., Campodonico, F., & Oliva, D. (2009a). A wheelchair user with visual and intellectual disabilities managing simple orientation technology for indoor travel. *Journal of Visual Impairment and Blindness, 103*, 308–313.

Lancioni, G. E., Singh, N. N., O'Reilly, M. F., Sigafoos, J., Didden, R., Manfredi, F., Putignano, P., Stasolla, F., & Basili, G. (2009b). Fostering locomotor behavior of children with developmental disabilities: An overview of studies using treadmills and walkers with microswitches. *Research in Developmental Disabilities, 30*, 308–322.

Lancioni, G. E., Singh, N. N., O'Reilly, M. F., Sigafoos, J., Oliva, D., Smaldone, A., La Martire, M. L., Stasolla, F., Castagnaro, F., & Groeneweg, J. (2010). Promoting ambulation responses among children with multiple disabilities through walkers and microswitches with contingent stimuli. *Research in Developmental Disabilities, 31*, 811–816.

Lee, L.-L., Watson, M. C., Mulvaney, C. A., Tsai, C.-C., & Lo, S.-F. (2010). The effect of walking intervention on blood pressure control: A systematic review. *International Journal of Nursing Studies, 47*, 1545–1561.

Liso, D. R. (2010). The effects of choice making on toy engagement in nonambulatory and partially ambulatory preschool students. *Topics in Early Childhood Special Education, 30*, 91–101.

Lloyd, M., Burghardt, A., Ulrich, D. A., & Angulo-Barroso, R. (2010). Physical activity and walking onset in infants with Down syndrome. *Adapted Physical Activity Quarterly, 27*, 1–16.

Looper, J., & Ulrich, D. A. (2010). Effect of treadmill training and supramalleolar orthosis use on motor skill development in infants with Down syndrome: A randomized clinical trial. *Physical Therapy, 90*, 382–390.

Lotan, M., Isakov, E., Kessel, S., & Merrick, J. (2004a). Physical fitness and functional ability of children with intellectual disability: Effects of short-term daily treadmill intervention. *The Scientific World, 4*, 449–457.

Lotan, M., Isakov, E., & Merrick, J. (2004b). Improving functional skills and physical fitness in children with Rett syndrome. *Journal of Intellectual Disability Research, 48*, 730–735.

Maher, C. A., Evans, K. A., Sprod, J. A., & Bostok, S. M. (2011). Factors influencing postural management for children with cerebral palsy in the special school setting. *Disability and Rehabilitation, 33*, 146–158.

Miltenberger, R. G. (2004). *Behavior modification: Principles and procedures* (3rd ed.). New York: Wadsworth.

Nolan, K. J., Savalia, K. K., Yarossi, M., & Elovic, E. P. (2010). Evaluation of a dynamic ankle foot orthosis in hemiplegic gait: A case report. *NeuroRehabilitation, 27*, 343–350.

Palisano, R. J., Tieman, B. L., Walter, S. D., Bartlett, D. J., Rosembaum, P. L., Russell, D., & Hanna, S. E. (2003). Effect of environmental setting on mobility methods of children with cerebral palsy. *Developmental Medicine and Child Neurology, 45*, 113–120.

Provost, B., Dieruf, K., Burtner, P. A., Phillips, J. P., Bernitsky-Beddingfield, A., Sullivan, K. J., Bowen, C. A., & Toser, L. (2007). Endurance and gait in children with cerebral palsy after intensive body weight-supported treadmill training. *Pediatric Physical Therapy, 19*, 2–10.

Richards, S. B., Taylor, R. L., Ramasamy, R., & Richards, R. Y. (1999). *Single subject research: Applications in educational and clinical settings*. New York: Wadsworth.

Russell, D., Rosenbaum, P., Avery, L., & Lane, M. (2002). *The gross motor function measure (GMFM-66 & GMFM-88) user's manual* (Clinics in developmental medicine, Vol. 159). London: Mac Keith Press.

Samuelsson, K., & Wressle, E. (2008). User satisfaction with mobility assistive devices: An important element in the rehabilitation process. *Disability and Rehabilitation, 30*, 551–558.

Sanders, E., Begnoche, D., & Pitetti, K. H. (2005). Effect of an intensive physical therapy program with partial body weight treadmill training on a 9 year-old child with spastic diplegic cerebral palsy. *Pediatric Physical Therapy, 17*, 82.

Schindl, M. R., Forstner, C., Kern, H., & Hesse, S. (2000). Treadmill training with partial body weight support in nonambulatory patients with cerebral palsy. *Archives of Physical Medicine and Rehabilitation, 81*, 301–306.

Schmidt, H., Werner, C., Bernhardt, R., Hesse, S., & Krüger, J. (2007). Gait rehabilitation machines based on programmable footplates. *Journal of Neuroengineering and Rehabilitation, 4*, 2.

Simard-Tremblay, E., Shevell, M., & Dagenais, L. (2010). Determinants of ambulation in children with spastic quadriplegic cerebral palsy: A population-based study. *Journal of Child Neurology, 25*, 669–673.

Storey, K. (1996). Social validation issues in social skills assessment. *International Journal of Disability, Development and Education, 43*, 167–174.

Strawbridge, L. A., Drnach, M., Sisson, L. A., & Van Hasselt, V. B. (1989). Behavioral therapy combined with physical therapy to promote walker use by a child with multiple handicaps. *Education and Training in Mental Retardation, 24*, 239–247.

Tieman, B., Palisano, R. J., Gracely, E. J., Rosenbaum, P., Chiarello, L. A., & O'Neil, M. (2004). Changes in mobility of children with cerebral palsy over time and across environmental settings. *Physical & Occupational Therapy in Pediatrics, 24*, 109–128.

Tsorlakis, N., Evaggelinou, C., Grouios, G., & Tsorbatzoudis, C. (2004). Effect of intensive neurodevelopmental treatment in gross motor function of children with cerebral palsy. *Developmental Medicine and Child Neurology, 46*, 740–745.

Ulrich, D. A., Ulrich, B. D., Angulo-Kinzler, R. M., & Yun, J. (2001). Treadmill training of infants with Down syndrome: Evidence-based developmental outcomes. *Pediatrics, 108*, e84.

Ulrich, D. A., Lloyd, M. C., Tiernan, C. W., Looper, J. E., & Angulo-Barroso, R. M. (2008). Effects of intensity of treadmill training on developmental outcomes and stepping in infants with Down syndrome: A randomized trial. *Physical Therapy, 88*, 114–122.

Van Gestel, L., Molenaers, G., Huenaerts, C., Seyler, J., & Desloovere, K. (2008). Effect of dynamic orthoses on gait: A retrospective control study in children with hemiplegia. *Developmental Medicine and Child Neurology, 50*, 63–67.

Vashdi, E., Hutzler, Y., & Roth, D. (2008). Compliance of children with moderate or severe intellectual disability to treadmill walking: A pilot study. *Journal of Intellectual Disability Research, 52*, 371–379.

Whittingham, K., Fahey, M., Rawicki, B., & Boyd, R. (2010). The relationship between motor abilities and early social development in a preschool cohort of children with cerebral palsy. *Research in Developmental Disabilities, 31*, 1346–1351.

Willoughby, K. L., Dodd, K. J., Shields, N., & Foley, S. (2010). Efficacy of partial body weight-supported treadmill training compared with overground walking practice for children with cerebral palsy: A randomized controlled trial. *Archives of Physical Medicine and Rehabilitation, 91*, 333–339.

Wu, J., Looper, J., Ulrich, B. D., Ulrich, D. A., & Angulo-Barroso, R. M. (2007). Exploring effects of different treadmill interventions on walking onset and gait patterns in infants with Down syndrome. *Developmental Medicine and Child Neurology, 49*, 839–845.

Wu, J., Ulrich, D. A., Looper, J., Tiernan, C. W., & Angulo-Barroso, R. M. (2008). Strategy adoption and locomotor adjustment in obstacle clearance of newly walking toddlers with Down syndrome after different treadmill interventions. *Experimental Brain Research, 186*, 261–272.

Zwicker, J. G., & Mayson, T. A. (2010). Effectiveness of treadmill training in children with motor impairments: An overview of systematic reviews. *Pediatric Physical Therapy, 22*, 361–377.

Chapter 7
Assistive Technology for Reducing Problem Behavior

Abstract In this chapter, we describe the use of assistive technology to treat or support individuals with severe/profound and multiple disabilities who engage in problem behavior. This chapter consists of two major sections. First, we begin with an overview of the nature of problem behavior with this population. As such, we will attempt to define problem behavior and describe what it looks like, examine the extent of these difficulties with this population, and finally outline strategies of clinical assessment and categorization of such behavior. Second, we present a selective overview of published peer-reviewed research that has examined the use of assistive technology to reduce such problem behaviors with this population. This overview of the assistive technology intervention research is presented according to the various categories of problem behavior outlined in the first major section of this chapter. Finally, we provide an overall summary of the use of assistive technology to reduce problem behavior and offer suggestions for future research in this area.

Introduction

Definition and Description of Problem Behavior

The definition and description of problem behavior with individuals with intellectual disabilities has and continues to receive an enormous amount of attention in the literature (Emerson and Einfeld 2011). While numerous definitions of problem behavior abound, these varieties can be distilled into two fundamental properties: behavior that is (a) harmful to the person's health and safety or to the health and safety of others sharing the person's environment and/or can (b) interfere with the person's access to regular community settings. This definition is purposefully broad. As such, it can accommodate an infinite number of types or topographies of behavior. This definition also allows for contextual sensitivity when defining problem

G.E. Lancioni et al., *Assistive Technology: Interventions for Individuals with Severe/Profound and Multiple Disabilities*, Autism and Child Psychopathology Series, DOI 10.1007/978-1-4614-4229-5_7,

Table 7.1 Frequently reported topographies of problem behavior

Aggression	Self-injury	Stereotyped behavior[a]	Property destruction
Hit with hand	Head hit open hand	Hand flapping	Break windows
Hit with object	Head hit fist	Body rocking	Tear materials
Kick	Eye poke	Finger flicking	Break chairs
Scratch	Head hit object	Object manipulation[b]	Rip clothes
Bite	Pinch/scratch	Head weaving	Breaks electronics
Pull hair	Pica[c]	Pacing	
Pinch	Bruxism[d]		
Verbal abuse	Hand mouthing		

[a]These patterns of stereotyped responding do not typically produce injury to self
[b]Using everyday toys/utensils in a repetitive nonfunctional manner
[c]Eating inedible objects
[d]Teeth grinding

behavior. For example, a behavior such as masturbation is problematic in a grocery store but may be acceptable in the privacy of one's bedroom.

Problem behavior with persons with intellectual disabilities is typically described in terms of three broad categories including aggression, self-injury, and property destruction (Emerson et al. 2001; Oliver et al. 1987; Sigafoos et al. 2003). Non-self-injurious stereotyped patterns of responding are sometimes added as a fourth category (Lancioni et al. 2012). Aggression is a deliberate act of violence or threat of such against another. Self-injury involves behaviors that produce harm to the self. Self-injurious behaviors can be dramatic and dangerous such as banging one's head against an object or they may seem innocuous at first glance but produce deleterious outcomes in the long term (e.g., hand mouthing). Property destruction involves breaking and damaging items and materials in the immediate environment. Non-self-injurious stereotyped movements involve repetitive nonfunctional body movements such as head weaving. Such behaviors are problematic in that they may interfere with adaptive programming and may be stigmatizing in community settings. While there are a wide variety of different topographies of problem behavior reported under each of these categories, some frequently reported topographies are illustrated in Table 7.1.

Extent of Problem Behavior with Individuals with Severe/ Profound and Multiple Disabilities

Despite the enormous amount of published research dedicated to the study of prevalence of problem behavior with this population, the picture remains unclear (Cooper et al. 2009a, b; Sigafoos et al. 2003). Prevalence estimates of problem behavior for the broader population of intellectual disability have ranged from as low as 2 % to a high of over 40 % and even as high as 70 % in some studies. This discrepancy in findings reflects differences in populations sampled and data collection methods

(Sigafoos et al. 2003). For example, studies conducted with institutionalized populations usually reflect a higher prevalence of problem behavior (e.g., Saloviita 2000). However, individuals may be admitted or remain in institutions for the very reason that they engage in severe problem behavior. Hence, such samples may be biased toward finding a high prevalence of such behaviors. More accurate estimates of prevalence can be accomplished through sampling whole populations (e.g., Emerson et al. 2001; Qureshi and Alborz 1992; Sigafoos et al. 1994). Methods of collecting information on problem behavior have also varied across studies. Some studies have conducted mailed surveys while others have involved interviews with caregivers and still others have used combinations of questionnaires and interview. As a result, definitions of problem behavior and the depth of information gleaned differ across prevalence studies. Despite these discrepancies across studies, Sigafoos et al. (2003) analyzed the whole population prevalence studies and surmised that approximately 15 % of individuals with intellectual disabilities engage in problem behavior.

When we begin to examine the extent of problem behavior with individuals with severe/profound multiple disabilities, the water becomes even murkier. Very few studies have attempted to examine the extent of problem behavior with this population, and many of these studies have looked at subgroups of this population such as people with severe disabilities and autism (e.g., Chadwick et al. 2008; Murphy et al. 2005) or profound multiple disabilities (e.g., Poppes et al. 2010). It is difficult to get a clear picture as to the prevalence of different types of challenging behavior in some of these studies. For example, Murphy et al. (2005) report *aggression*, *rebellion*, *uncooperative*, *temper tantrums*, and *public behavior* as separate variables. On the face of it, these variables may have considerable overlap (variations of aggression) and combined might produce a broader picture as to the overall prevalence of aggression with this sample. The research by Chadwick et al. (2008) primarily focuses on risk factors associated with challenging behavior for individuals with severe disabilities.

The most comprehensive overview of prevalence of problem behavior with individuals with severe/profound multiple disabilities was conducted by Poppes et al. (2010). In this study, the authors used the Behavior Problem Inventory (BPI) (Rojahn et al. 2001) to assess prevalence of self-injury, stereotypy, and aggressive behavior in a sample of 181 individuals with profound intellectual and multiple disabilities. They also examined the presence of sensory (e.g., visual impairment) and health problems (e.g., epilepsy) with the sample. Again, this study has limitations for our purpose as it is limited to individuals with profound multiple disabilities (not severe disabilities). Additionally, the entire sample was obtained from institutional settings. As mentioned earlier, institutional samples tend to reflect higher levels of problem behavior. However, it may be difficult to obtain a large sample of individuals with profound disabilities residing in community settings in any case. The results of this study show that 82 % of the sample engaged in self-injury and stereotypy, respectively, while 45 % engaged in aggressive behavior. These are staggering prevalence figures when we compare prevalence of problem behavior to the broader population of intellectual disability described earlier in this section (i.e., 15 %). In an interesting addendum to this research, Poppes et al. (2010) note that Rojahn et al.

(2001) administered the BPI to a sample with broader levels of disability and produced contrasting results. In the Rojahn et al. findings, self-injury, stereotypy, and aggression occurred with 43 %, 54 %, and 43 % of their sample, respectively. This comparison of results seems to indicate that self-injury and stereotypy may be more prevalent among persons with profound/multiple disabilities.

Another interesting finding of the Poppes et al. (2010) study was that a large percentage of participants suffered from sensory and health problems. Visual and auditory problems were experienced by 73 % and 39 % of the sample, respectively. Bowel and abdominal problems were experienced by 78 % while 66 % suffered from epilepsy. Other health problems experienced by a large proportion of this sample included psychiatric, sleep, and respiratory disorders. Health and sensory problems may predispose and/or exacerbate challenging behaviors such as self-injury and aggression with this population (Carr and Smith 1995; Lancioni et al. 1999; Sigafoos et al. 2003).

Clinical Assessment and Categorization of Problem Behavior

Thus far in this chapter, we have defined what we mean by problem behavior and described the most common types or topographies of problem behavior with individuals with severe/profound and multiple disabilities. We then attempted to understand how pervasive problem behaviors are with this population by examining the prevalence of problem behavior. In this section, we are going to talk about the clinical assessment of problem behavior. Clinical assessment is not interested in what problem behavior looks like, as topography does not dictate what the most effective treatment might be for such behavior. Instead clinical assessment of problem behavior focuses on the function of such behaviors. Understanding the function of problem behavior entails an examination of the reinforcing or stimulating consequences produced by the problem behavior. Clinical assessments designed to identify the function of problem behavior usually take the form of rating scales, observational protocols, or analogue functional analyses. It is now accepted practice to conduct some form of assessment of the function of problem behavior prior to selecting an intervention strategy (Lancioni et al. 2012). Two of these clinical assessment tools are described below to illustrate.

The *Questions about Behavioral Function* (QABF) is a rating scale that consists of a series of structured questions about the possible functions of problem behavior (Matson et al. 1999; Matson and Wilkins 2009; Paclawskyj et al. 2000; Singh et al. 2009). The questionnaire is designed to be answered by staff that works closely with the person with problem behavior. It can be administered in a short period of time (about 30 min). This rating scale consists of a 25- or a briefer 19-item questionnaire that is designed to identify contexts under which challenging behavior is more likely to occur. A total of five contexts are probed using the QABF including whether the problem behavior is more likely when the person is (a) left alone (indicating that the problem behavior is self-stimulatory or stereotyped in nature), (b) engaged in difficult tasks (indicating that problem behavior is a form of protest in order to avoid or escape demanding tasks), (c) denied access to preferred items (indicating that problem behavior is an attempt to gain access to preferred items), (d) in a social context where attention is diverted away from him or her (indicating that problem behavior is an attempt to access social attention from others), and (e) suffering from physical discomfort (indicating that problem behavior may be a response to some form of physical distress/pain).

The *analogue functional analysis* is by far the most researched clinical assessment technique to identify function of problem behavior (Hanley et al. 2003; Iwata et al. 1982/1994). In an analogue functional analysis, the person is repeatedly exposed to a series of social situations that are analogous to commonly experienced social contexts. Each social situation usually lasts anywhere from 5 to 20 min and is repeated in a random or semirandom fashion, thereby demonstrating experimental control. Targeted problem behavior is measured during these social situations. If problem behavior occurs more frequently in one or more social situations relative to others, then it is inferred that consequences in those particular social situations are maintaining problem behavior. The social situations examined in the analogue functional analysis mirror many of the contexts identified in the QABF.

Three of the social conditions of the analogue functional analysis will be described (attention, demand, alone) to give the reader an impression of how such an assessment is conducted. In the *attention condition*, the person is placed in a room with a therapist. The therapist appears busy (often writing or reading) and does not interact with the person unless problem behavior occurs at which point the therapist delivers statements of concern ("Don't do that. You'll hurt yourself"). The therapist then returns to reading or writing and does not interact with the person again unless problem behavior occurs. If there is a high frequency of problem behavior in the attention condition relative to other conditions, then we can infer that problem behavior is maintained by access to attention from others. In the *demand condition*, the therapist presents tasks to the person that they have difficulty completing. Tasks used in this condition are often selected from the person's individualized education plan and have not yet been mastered. Instruction is continued on these tasks throughout the condition unless problem behavior occurs at which point the task is removed for a minimum time period or until problem behavior desists at which point the task is reintroduced. Instruction again continues until problem behavior occurs once more. If there is a high frequency of problem behavior in the demand condition relative to other conditions, then we can infer that problem behavior is maintained by escape from task demands. Finally, in the *alone condition*, the person is placed in a room on their own. Typically, there are no stimulating items (e.g., toys, books) available in the room in order to simulate a barren environment. No consequences are programmed for problem behavior in this condition. High levels of problem behavior in the alone condition relative to other conditions indicate that problem behavior is self-stimulatory or stereotyped in nature.

The above descriptions of the QABF and analogue functional analysis present examples of assessments from a wide variety of interviews, rating scales, and observational techniques that can be used by the clinician to identify the function of problem behavior. The common thrust of all these clinical assessment techniques is to identify contexts in which problem behavior is more likely. In particular, these assessments are geared to identify consequences that maintain problem behavior such as self-stimulation, escape from aversive demands, access to tangible items, or attention. Some of these assessments also include attempts to identify health and other biological variables that may predispose the person to challenging behavior (e.g., QABF).

Information derived from these assessments is then used to tailor interventions to treat the problem behavior. For example, if a person's problem behavior is shown to be self-stimulatory in nature, then one intervention option might be to provide the person with similar but appropriate forms of alternative stimulation and possibly teach the person to request this stimulation. Persons whose problem behavior is maintained by escape from demanding situations might be taught to communicate for brief breaks from the task and/or to request help with said task. Those whose problem behavior is maintained by access to tangible or attention may be taught appropriate means to request tangibles or attention. Overall, we can see that the results of such assessments allow for the clinician to adopt a positive educational approach to the treatment of problem behavior by replacing such behavior with adaptive alternative responses (Sigafoos et al. 2003).

In the next section of this chapter, we will outline interventions using assistive technology to reduce problem behavior with individuals with severe/profound and multiple disabilities. These interventions will be discussed according to whether they were used to treat problem behavior that is maintained by access to attention or tangible items, escape from demands, or are self-stimulatory in nature.

Overview of Assistive Technology Used to Treat Problem Behavior

In this section, we present a selective overview of intervention studies using assistive technology designed to treat problem behavior with individuals with severe/profound and multiple disabilities. The studies are grouped according to the clinical classifications (demand, tangible, attention, and self-stimulation). In the last decade or so, it has become accepted clinical practice to use some form of clinical assessment/judgment as to what might be maintaining problem behavior and then use this information to build an intervention (Kahng et al. 2002). For each clinical classification (e.g., attention, demand), we provide a detailed description of one or more cases from the intervention studies. This includes a detailed description of the participants involved, topography of problem behavior, type of technology used, and experimental protocols (e.g., instruction, maintenance, and generalization of treatment effects).

Assistive Technology to Treat Problem Behavior Maintained by Escape

A small number of studies have used assistive technology to treat problem behavior maintained by escape from demands (e.g., Durand 1993, 1999; Steege et al. 1990). Preintervention assessment of the function of problem behavior was conducted in these studies. Several layers of functional assessment were utilized across the studies including interviews with caregivers (parents, teachers) as to the nature, extent, and history of the behaviors; questionnaires such as the Motivation Assessment Scale (Durand and Crimmins 1992); and analogue functional analysis. Following these assessments, an augmentative communication device was selected, and participants were taught to use this technology to communicate a desire to terminate demands. Problem behavior is typically ignored during these instructional sessions. The goal of these interventions was to teach the person to use the augmentative communication device to escape or terminate demands, thus making the escape-maintained problem behavior unnecessary.

For example, Steege et al. (1990) report an intervention with Dennis, a 6-year-old boy who was nonverbal, was nonambulatory (confined to a wheelchair), and was diagnosed with profound intellectual disabilities. He possessed no independent communication skills and was dependent on others for all self-care needs. He was referred to a hospital inpatient unit because of problem behavior, and intervention took place in a classroom that was located in this inpatient unit. Dennis engaged in self-injury consisting of hand, wrist, and arm biting. This self-injury, while present since Dennis was 2 years old, had recently increased in severity and frequency, causing open wounds on his hands and arms. Interviews with Dennis's mother and teacher indicated that self-injury was most problematic when he was engaged in self-care routines (e.g., face washing, hair combing, tooth brushing). These self-care tasks were subsequently included in the demand conditions of an analogue functional analysis. Results of the analogue functional analysis indicated that self-injury occurred almost exclusively during the demand condition for Dennis. The results of the analogue functional analysis therefore indicated that Dennis engaged in self-injury primarily to escape self-care tasks. The augmentative communication device used in this study included a contact (pressure) microswitch (15 cm × 15 cm) which when pressed operated a tape recorder which played the message "Stop!" The intervention consisted of teaching Dennis to press the switch during grooming routines producing a removal of the task for 10 s. He was physically guided to press the switch by the therapist or he could independently press the switch. In either case, the pressing of the switch produced removal of the task for 10 s. If Dennis engaged in self-injury during instruction, the task was continued (he was not allowed to self-injure and was physically guided through the task). This intervention produced a rapid decrease in self-injury with a concomitant increase of prompted and independent use of the augmentative communication device. Dennis was further evaluated at 6 months following the intervention, and these follow-up results remained positive with high levels of independent use of the communication device and low levels of self-injury.

Assistive Technology to Treat Problem Behavior Maintained by Access to Tangible Items

As with demand-related problem behavior, there are a limited number of examples of using assistive technology to treat tangibly maintained problem behavior with persons with severe/profound multiple disabilities (e.g., Durand 1993, 1999). Preintervention assessment was conducted initially to identify the nature of problem behavior. This assessment process consisted of general interviews with significant caregivers to identify severity, nature, and context of the problem behavior. These general interviews were then followed with rating scales such as the Motivation Assessment Scale (Durand and Crimmins 1992) and in some cases analogue functional analysis to identify reinforcing consequences for the problem behavior. Following these assessments, new communicative responses were selected. These new responses would serve the same function of problem behavior (access the same tangible items that problem behavior produced) and eventually come to replace such problem behavior. Augmentative communication devices were also selected based on the nature of the problem behavior. Such devices needed to be simple enough for the participant to operate efficiently and effectively given the severity of their disabilities. Considerations with regard to the robustness of the device were also addressed given the nature of some of the problem behavior with some of these participants (i.e., aggression and property destruction). Following these assessments, the participant was taught to use the augmentative device to communicate a desire to access tangible items. Problem behavior was ignored during instructional sessions (did not result in access to tangible items as before). The goal of these interventions was to teach the participant to use the augmentative communication device to access the desired tangible items and thus make problem behavior unnecessary in such circumstances.

For example, Durand (1993) describes an intervention with Joshua, a 3-year-old boy with severe intellectual disability. Joshua lived at home with his parents and attended a public preschool. He had no formal communication system and was reported as having a language age of 15 months. He was capable of feeding himself and was cooperative with self-help skills routines. No physical disabilities were described. His parents were interviewed regarding problem behavior and reported that it occurred primarily around meal and snack time. Parents also noted that he was very fond of food. Joshua's problem behavior consisted of tantrums and included crying, screaming, and hitting others. His parents described his problem behavior as being frequent. A teacher and assistant teacher administered the Motivation Assessment Scale (Durand and Crimmins 1992), and the results of this functional assessment indicated that Joshua's behavior was tangibly maintained (access to food). Intervention then was targeted at those times when behavior was problematic (mealtimes), and the communication response selected to replace the problem behavior was "I want more." A Wolf™ communication device was used with Joshua. The author notes that this device was selected based on cost and durability considerations (it can withstand some physical abuse). The Wolf™ uses synthesized speech and is activated using a pressure pad. Joshua was then taught to use the communication device to signal that he wanted more food during mealtimes. Parents and teachers used a combination of instructional prompts such as physically guiding Joshua's hand to press the device during meals. All activations of the device were reinforced with food while problem behavior was ignored during training. Training continued for 2 weeks until Joshua used the device on five consecutive occasions without any instructional prompts. Joshua continued to independently use the device to request food following training while his problem behavior remained at very low levels. An interesting addition to this study is that the author measured expressions of affect during intervention. Affect included measures of positive facial expression and smiling. Joshua's positive affect increased dramatically during mealtimes with the introduction of the augmentative communication system. This additional measurement of affect adds further to the veracity of using augmentative communication devices to replace challenging behavior with this population.

Assistive Technology to Treat Problem Behavior Maintained by Access to Attention

Again, there are a limited number of studies demonstrating the use of assistive technology to treat attention-maintained problem behavior with the severe/profound multiple disability population (Durand 1993, 1999). The process of assessment, device selection, and general intervention protocols are similar to the case studies described with escape-maintained and tangible-maintained problem behavior above. In general, the intervention process begins with a detailed unstructured interview with caregivers to clarify the nature and contexts in which problem behavior occurs. Following the unstructured interview, rating scales are then administered. These scales are designed to clarify the function (consequences produced) of the problem behavior. In all cases reviewed for attention-maintained behavior, the participants were finally assessed using the analogue functional analysis technique to verify the maintaining consequences for their problem behavior. Following this assessment process, an augmentative communication device was selected. Issues considered when selecting the device included ease of use (matched to the intellectual and physical disabilities of the participant), robustness (device needed to be able to withstand some abuse as problem behavior included aggression with most participants), and cost (device had to be cost-effective). The device was then programmed with a vocalization that would elicit attention from caregivers. The participant is then taught to use the device to solicit attention while problem behavior is ignored. The goal of these interventions is to eventually replace problem behavior with appropriate responding via the augmentative communication device.

For example, Durand (1999) reports an intervention with Ron, a 9-year-old boy diagnosed with autism and severe intellectual disability (reported language and mental age of 45 and 38 months, respectively). He was reported to use some words, but these were not used in a contextually appropriate manner. He did not speak when prompted. His problem behavior was aggression and was defined as hitting forcefully with his hands. Ron was described as being very aggressive and targeted family, teachers, and fellow students. Assessment and intervention was carried out in Ron's classroom with subsequent generalization probes conducted in the community by his teachers. The Motivation Assessment Scale (Durand and Crimmins 1992) was completed by his teacher and teacher aide, and then an analogue functional analysis was conducted. The results of both the rating scale and analogue functional analysis indicated that Ron's aggression was maintained by access to attention from others. Following these assessments, the author (V. M. Durand) met with parents, teacher, and an assistive technology professional to agree upon an augmentative communication device that would be appropriate for Ron. The Introtalker™ was selected as it requires little force to press the keypad, it is a relatively robust device, and it uses digitized speech that is highly intelligible to the listener. The Introtalker™ was programmed with one phrase to request attention, "Would you help me with this?" Ron was then taught to use his device to request attention in the classroom. Instruction continued for approximately 4 weeks. Throughout the school day, Ron was prompted (physical, gestural, and verbal prompts) to use his device to gain attention. Prompts were gradually faded (teaching staff waited between 3 and 5 s before delivering a prompt) to promote independence. Instruction continued until Ron used his device independently in the appropriate context on five consecutive occasions. This training in the classroom lasted approximately 4 weeks. Ron's aggression was virtually eliminated in the classroom with the introduction of the communication device. Corresponding with the decrease of aggression, there was a concomitant increase in spontaneous communication for Ron. A very interesting extension of this work was that generalization of the intervention to a regular community setting was assessed. Ron enjoyed visiting a local magazine store. Prior to the intervention, his aggression attempts were measured in the store. The teacher was present to block any attempts at aggression toward customers and staff. Aggression was quite high in the store prior to the intervention. Ron was again escorted to the store once he had reached independent performance with his communication device in the classroom. Ron independently used his device to request attention, and aggression was reduced dramatically in the magazine store. Additionally, store staff responded to 100 % of his requests for help/attention. In sum, Ron learned to use his communication device independently in the classroom, and he spontaneously generalized the use of this device to a community setting. Problem behavior was virtually eliminated in both contexts.

Assistive Technology to Treat Self-stimulatory Problem Behavior

The majority of published research that has used assistive technology to treat problem behavior with individuals with severe/profound multiple disabilities has focused on the treatment of self-stimulatory behavior (see Lancioni et al. 2009 for a comprehensive review). This emphasis on intervention with this type of problem behavior should be expected given our discussion of prevalence earlier in this chapter. As we may recall, the Poppes et al. (2010) study reported that 82 % of their sample of individuals with profound multiple disabilities engaged in self-injury and stereotypy. These types of self-stimulatory behavior patterns do not serve a communicative function (such as escape from aversive situations, attention from others, etc.). The positive consequences that motivate such behavior are best considered to be endogenous. As such, we do not see externally directed problem behavior (i.e., aggression and property destruction) addressed with these interventions but rather a focus on self-injurious and stereotyped behaviors (see Table 7.1). This is not to say that self-injurious or stereotyped behaviors cannot serve a social-communicative function. However, in this body of work, it was determined via prior interview of significant others, casual observation, or analogue functional analysis that the behaviors in question did not serve a social function (e.g., Kennedy and Souza 1995; Lancioni et al. 2007).

A variety of assistive technologies have been included in programs to treat self-stimulatory problem behavior such as tilt, pressure, and optic microswitches. These microswitches have often been adapted to capture minimal levels of motor behavior with the participants in these studies (e.g., foot, back, tongue, head responses). The intervention studies themselves can be categorized into three general types of intervention strategy: (1) microswitches linked to a self-stimulatory response that produces a prompt to reduce the response, (2) microswitches that produce positive stimulation when an adaptive alternative behavior to self-stimulation occurs, and (3) microswitch clusters where an adaptive response (monitored by one microswitch) produces positive stimulation only when the self-stimulatory response (monitored by the second microswitch) does not occur. Examples from each of these three categories of microswitch intervention are described below to illustrate.

As an example of category 1 above, Lancioni et al. (2005b) evaluated the use of a microswitch to deliver prompts to reduce persistent tongue protrusion. The participant involved was a 39-year-old woman who was reported to be functioning in the severe to profound range of intellectual disability. She attended a day activity center where she engaged in simple activities such as sorting objects and listening to music. She possessed no intelligible speech but could understand simple directions such as to withdraw her tongue. The behavior targeted for intervention was tongue protrusion and was defined as the tongue sticking out of the lower lip. Observations prior to intervention or when the intervention was withdrawn demonstrated that she engaged in tongue protrusion at or above 50 % of the time. Tongue protrusion also seemed to occur independent of the social context. Assistive technology consisted of (a) an optic sensor (miniphotocell) attached to the lower lip using medical tape, (b) a signal transmission box, and (c) a Walkman. Both the Walkman and signal transmission box were placed in a pocket of the woman's clothing. The optic sensor was activated when tongue protrusion occurred, and this activated the Walkman that delivered a phrase to prompt the woman to withdraw her tongue. Tongue protrusion was virtually eliminated with use of this technology. However, each time the technology was withdrawn, protrusion returned to prior levels (approximately 50 % of the time). The authors note that while the optic sensor location might be too intrusive for use over extended periods of time, it might be valuable to consider fading the technology perhaps to phrases intermittently delivered by the Walkman alone. This technology therefore served to automatically prompt the woman to withdraw her tongue each time protrusion occurred. It proved to be highly effective and virtually eliminated self-stimulatory behavior for sessions of anywhere between 20 and 60 min.

An example of a category 2 intervention is illustrated in Lancioni et al. (2011). In this study, the authors examined the use of microswitch technology to treat drooling, a prevalent difficulty with individuals with severe intellectual and physical disabilities. The authors note that drooling is typically associated with some physical difficulty such as overproduction of saliva or mouth malocclusion rather than serving a social function. To illustrate, one of the participants in this study was Graham, a 46-year-old man with severe to profound intellectual disability. He possessed residual vision due to optic atrophy and suffered from severe (partially controlled) epilepsy. He had some echolalic speech and could perform some simple occupational tasks such as collecting and matching objects. He attended day care rehabilitation where he received physiotherapy and was engaged in simple leisure activities. Drooling was reported to be always present. Graham seemed to overproduce saliva, rarely swallowed or tried to clean his mouth spontaneously. The assistive technology consisted of a special napkin placed around his neck. The lower half of the napkin was thick and absorbent and could be replaced when wet. Graham was to use this thicker section of the napkin to wipe his mouth. Two pressure sensors were embedded in the thick section of the napkin. A mouth-wiping response (bringing the lower part of the napkin to the mouth and pushing the napkin to the mouth) would activate at least one of these pressure sensors. The activation of a pressure sensor in the napkin triggered a microprocessor that in turn activated an MP3 player. The microprocessor and MP3 device were small items that were housed in the upper part of the napkin. Thus, when Graham wiped his mouth, he received 10 s of highly preferred music and songs. This music and songs were systematically identified using a preference assessment prior to the study. Once the 10 s of music elapsed, Graham could again wipe his mouth and activate the music once more. Eventually, additional music was added to the MP3 device (approximately 10 s of additional but less preferred music) to increase the intervals between mouth wipes with Graham (a lower frequency of mouth wiping looked more socially acceptable but continued to be effective in terms of eliminating drooling). Chin wetness and mouth wiping were measured when the technology was present and absent. Results of the research demonstrated that assistive technology resulted in substantial increases in mouth wiping and virtually eliminated chin wetness. The technology continued to be effective for controlling drooling at a 3-month follow-up. This research demonstrates that simple assistive technology (pressure microswitch, microprocessor, MP3 device) can be used to deliver positive stimulation that established a routine behavior pattern (mouth wiping) to control the effects of drooling.

Several examples of category 3 (use of multiple microswitches) will be presented. The reason why we dwell on category 3 interventions is because these interventions are clinically the most significant of the microswitch technologies used to treat self-stimulatory behavior with this population. As mentioned above and as discussed in the final section of this chapter, such combined microswitch technologies serve a dual purpose of increasing adaptive responding while simultaneously managing/reducing self-stimulatory responding.

Our first example of using multiple microswitches (category 3) to treat problem behavior can be found in Lancioni et al. (2007). As mentioned above, microswitch clusters usually involve one microswitch that is used to access positive stimulation when problem behavior (monitored by a second microswitch) does not occur. This combination of microswitches is valuable as it allows for the learning of adaptive responding while simultaneously controlling or reducing problem behavior (Lancioni et al. 2009). Lancioni et al. (2007) used a microswitch cluster to treat hand mouthing and eye poking for a 12-year-old boy. The boy was in the profound range of intellectual disability. He suffered from congenital cerebropathy with spastic tetraparesis, possessed minimal residual vision, and suffered from seizures. He had no speech, consistent communication, or self-help skills and was confined to a wheelchair. The authors report that hand mouthing (bringing the fingers or other parts of the hand into or over the mouth) and eye poking (placing the fingers into or over the eye) occurred independent of social contingencies. Both eye poking and hand mouthing were monitored by optical microswitches (photocells) that were held to the right side of the boy's face via light wires, and these wires were in turn attached to a headband (worn during sessions). The boy's left arm did not function—hence the reason for the positioning of the photocells at the right side of the head. The adaptive response consisted of repeated lifting and shaking of the right foot (while seated in a wheelchair), and this activated a motion microswitch attached to the foot. The adaptive response produced 8 s of pleasant stimulation (determined via a prior preference assessment) and consisted of music, recorded voices of favorite persons, light displays, and vibratory stimulation. Microswitch responses were inputted to a control system, and this system recorded all three responses including adaptive responding in the absence of problem behavior. Eventually, the boy could access pleasant stimulation via the foot response but only when problem behavior did not occur. For example, if the boy attempted to eye poke or hand mouth while pleasant stimulation was occurring, then this was recorded by the optic microswitch(s) at the head, and pleasant stimulation was immediately interrupted. In other words, the boy could only access pleasant stimulation when he did not engage in hand mouthing and eye poking. The results of the study demonstrate substantial decreases in problem behavior with concomitant increases in foot responses. This intervention model is posited by the authors as a form of self-determination whereby the boy learned to control his problem behavior in order to access alternative pleasurable consequences via the adaptive response.

In a second example of category 3, Lancioni et al. (2010) implemented a microswitch intervention to reduce dystonic stretching of one or both arms either forward or sideward for Glen, a 5-year-old boy with a diagnosis of severe to profound intellectual disability. He was diagnosed with encephalopathy that was due to premature birth and perinatal hypoxia, and he also presented with spastic tetraparesis combined with dystonic movements. He spent most of his day in a wheelchair. He possessed no speech or means of communication, and his vision was severely impaired (he was reported to see relatively large objects within 1 m and at the center of the visual field). Glen lived at home with his parents and attended a day activity center that focused on physiotherapy and general stimulation goals.

Dystonic stretching is a relatively prevalent behavior pattern in individuals with multiple disabilities and can interfere with ongoing habilitation efforts. However, until this study, no research had attempted to reduce this problem behavior with this population. In essence, such patterns of behavior were seen as an essential characteristic of the disability and not as behaviors that were amenable to change.

The intervention consisted of Glen manipulating five to seven objects that were placed in an open box in front of him (base of box 37 cm × 27 cm and 10 cm high). The items placed in the box included such preferred items as favorite toys. These items were loosely tied to the bottom of the box. Adaptive responding for Glen consisted of manipulating these objects (by placing both hands in the box). This response was deemed adaptive as it was incompatible with dystonic arm stretching. In terms of microswitches, there were a number of microswitches placed in the box (including optic and tilt microswitches) that were placed under and on the objects. Manipulation of the objects activated the microswitches and produced preferred stimulation (these preferred stimuli were identified prior to the intervention using a stimulus preference screening approach). Preferred stimulation included music, familiar voices, vibratory input, and light displays for about 8 s contingent on manipulation of any of the items in the box. The second component of the microswitch cluster consisted of magnetic watch-like sensors attached to both wrists. These sensors detected the removal of one or both arms from the box (any distance greater than 10 cm for 2 s or more). Arm removal from the box produced termination of the preferred stimulation. Arm removal rather than dystonic arm movements was targeted for intervention as it was considered a precursor to dystonic arm movements. The effectiveness of this intervention was evaluated using an ABAB design. In the A phase, manipulation of the objects in the box did not activate microswitches to produce positive stimulation nor did removal of arms from the box produce termination of stimulation. In the B phase, microswitches produced the consequences described above. High levels of object manipulation (and therefore low levels of dystonic arm stretching) occurred in the B phases of the research. These findings indicate that this microswitch cluster was effective in controlling dystonic arm stretching for Glen.

A final example of a microswitch cluster was developed by Lancioni et al. (2008) to manage head control in persons with multiple disabilities. Poor head control (e.g., head forward tilting) can be considered a problem behavior as it interferes with educational programming and can have deleterious consequences on physical condition (such as breathing, muscle tone, etc.). As head tilting occurs almost continuously and in the absence of social contingencies for those affected, it would appear that such behavior is automatic in nature. In a series of case studies, Lancioni and colleagues have demonstrated that appropriate head control can be accomplished during active engagement sessions using microswitch cluster technology (e.g., Lancioni et al. 2004, 2005a, 2008). Lancioni et al. (2008) present the case example of Sid, a 7-year-old boy with encephalopathy, spastic tetraparesis, and severe to profound intellectual disability. He was confined to a wheelchair and had little hand, arm, and leg movement coupled with minimal trunk control. His head tended to tilt forward constantly. He had typical hearing but suffered from minimal residual vision. Sid lived at home with his parents and attended a day facility that focused on physiotherapy and stimulation. The adaptive response selected for Sid was foot lifting, and a tilt microswitch was attached to his leg in order to capture this response. A tilt microswitch was also attached to Sid's head via a headband. The head microswitch was activated when the head was upright and deactivated when his head was tilted. Sid was first taught to use the foot-lifting response to access preferred stimuli such as music, noises, chimes, television clips, and a variety of vibratory inputs. These preferred stimuli had been identified for Sid via a preference assessment screening procedure prior to the study. Activating the foot microswitch produced 8 s of a selection of these preferred stimuli. Once Sid had consolidated the foot-lifting response to access preferred stimuli, he was then required to hold his head upright (monitored by the second tilt microswitch) while making the foot-lifting response in order to access preferred stimulation. If his head tilted, then preferred stimulation did not occur or was immediately terminated. Results of this study show that Sid was able to learn to access the preferred stimuli via the foot-lifting response while keeping his head in an upright position.

Summary and Suggestions for Future Research

In this chapter, we examined the use of assistive technology to treat problem behavior for individuals with severe/profound and multiple disabilities. Problem behavior was defined broadly as any behavior that persistently interferes with the health and safety of the individual or others and/or limits successful community inclusion. Problem behaviors were broadly categorized as aggression, stereotyped behavior, self-injury, and property destruction. While prevalence of problem behavior with individuals with severe/profound multiple disabilities requires further research, it does seem that a large percentage of this population engage in such behavior. Problem behavior seems more likely with this population than with other individuals with developmental disabilities. Individuals with severe/profound multiple disabilities seem particularly prone to engage in self-injurious and stereotyped patterns of behavior. For the purposes of developing clinical interventions, problem behavior is assessed in terms of its functions or what outcomes it produces for the individual. The typical functions of problem behavior include gaining attention or tangible items, escaping demands, or are self-stimulatory in nature. Clinical interventions are tailored to the function of problem behavior, and we examined clinical interventions utilizing assistive technology to treat problem behavior across escape, tangible, attention, and self-stimulatory functions with this population.

Our selective review of the intervention research showed very positive outcomes in terms of using assistive technology to treat problem behavior with individuals with severe/profound multiple disabilities. In fact, all studies reviewed demonstrated a virtual elimination of problem behavior when the intervention was introduced. Interventions were successful across the range of functions including attention, tangible, demand, and self-stimulatory problem behavior. Additionally, the types of problem behavior could be considered as quite severe in many of these papers (eye poking, hitting, self-biting, tantrums) and chronic (present for several years for most of the participants). These findings illustrate that such interventions have robust utility. Additionally, while the number of studies reviewed is small, all studies utilized rigorous single-subject research design methodologies such as withdrawal and multiple-baseline (or probe) designs (Barlow et al. 2009). So while this is a small body of research, it does demonstrate replication of intervention effectiveness within participants (withdrawal design), across participants (multiple-baseline design), and finally across studies. Such experimental rigor allows us to be fairly confident about the findings of these studies.

A number of general points can be made regarding the assessment and instructional strategies used in these studies. First, all studies initially focused on an assessment of the status of the individual and function of the challenging behavior prior to designing an intervention using assistive technology. Some of the studies provide an extensive history of the disability and associated medical conditions (e.g., Lancioni et al. 2007, 2011). Such information can help with eliminating possible functions of problem behavior (e.g., drooling occurs because of physical malformation such as mouth malocclusion associated with the disability and therefore does not serve a social function) and determining the assistive technology to use based upon the physical abilities of the person. Other studies describe the severity of the challenging behavior (such as aggression and tantrums) and note that this influenced the selection of fairly robust assistive technology (because of the potential of abuse; Durand 1999). All studies that treated socially maintained problem behavior used a series of assessments including interview, questionnaire, and functional analysis to determine what consequences were maintaining problem behavior (Durand 1993, 1999; Steege et al. 1990). These functional assessment protocols were critical in determining subsequent interventions. Overall, the use of pretreatment assessments in all of these studies are in line with current consensus regarding pretreatment assessment of problem behavior and how these results should inform intervention selection (Sigafoos et al. 2003).

Second, studies that used assistive technology to treat socially maintained problem behavior (i.e., behavior maintained by access to attention, tangible items, or escape from demanding situations) used this assistive technology as part of a general functional communication intervention (FCT) protocol. FCT interventions are designed to replace problem behavior by teaching the person to access the desired outcomes (e.g., escape from a difficult task) using appropriate forms of communication. Participants learned to use a variety of assistive devices (e.g., Introtalker™, pressure microswitch and tape recorder, Wolf™ communication device) to produce an alternative appropriate response while the problem behavior was placed on extinction (Durand 1993, 1999; Steege et al. 1990). Participants were taught to use the devices to request desired consequences using relatively simple systems of instructional prompts such as physical guidance by a teacher, therapist, or parent to operate the switch. Many of the participants learned to independently operate the device in a relatively short period of time.

Third, studies that have employed assistive technology to treat self-stimulatory problem behavior have used a different approach to assessment and intervention. It is difficult, if not impossible, to isolate consequences that may be maintaining such patterns of responding. Earlier in this chapter, we hypothesized that consequences maintaining self-stimulatory behaviors may be endogenous in nature and so are not accessible to direct observation by a third party. Implementing an FCT model of treatment may therefore have limited success with many of these individuals. FCT is based on the premise that the individual is taught an appropriate alternative response to access the consequences maintaining problem behavior. In many of the studies reviewed, participants were first assessed to identify highly preferred items and activities (e.g., music, familiar voices, vibratory and light stimulation). These positive consequences were made contingent upon incompatible behavior (e.g., chin wiping for drooling responses) or an alternative adaptive behavior (e.g., foot lifting) when the problem behavior did not occur (e.g., eye poking). In all of these studies, the preferred items apparently overpowered whatever consequences were maintaining the self-stimulatory behavior as we see a virtual elimination of self-stimulatory behavior with concomitant increases in alternative and adaptive behaviors.

Fourth, the assistive technology used in interventions to treat self-stimulatory problem behavior was developed to meet the idiosyncratic needs of each of the participants. In comparison, commercially available technology was used in the interventions to treat socially mediated problem behavior. A number of reasons can be posited for developing and adapting technology in these studies. Participants with self-stimulatory behavior in these studies were functioning in the very severe and profound range of intellectual disability. Therefore, teaching them to independently utilize such devices as the Introtalker™ may have been an arduous or even impossible task. Participants also suffered from multiple physical disabilities and therefore often had minimal and idiosyncratic response patterns (see Lancioni et al. 2007 above). The assistive technology developed in these studies was intended to capture these minimal responses and establish a contingency between these adaptive responses and positive stimulation.

A number of considerations might be addressed in future research on the use of assistive technology to treat problem behavior with this population. While we only presented a selective overview of research on the use of technology to treat problem behavior with individuals with severe/profound disabilities, it is clear that there are a limited number of peer-reviewed empirical evaluations published on this topic. This is particularly true with regard to the use of assistive technology to treat socially mediated problem behavior. Future research should be conducted to replicate and extend the current body of research, particularly for socially mediated problem behavior. It is likely that individuals with multiple and profound disabilities also engage in socially mediated problem behavior. We could not find any research where communication devices such as an Introtalker™ were adapted using supplemental microswitch technology to treat socially mediated problem behavior.

In general, more research needs to be conducted on the use of assistive technology to treat such behaviors with this population.

In future research, the focus of intervention effectiveness should be extended beyond the ability of the technology and other intervention parameters to control problem behavior. This is not to say that there are no examples of generalization and maintenance of treatment effects and social validity measures in the studies reviewed. However, measures of generalization, maintenance, and validity should be incorporated as a routine agenda within all such research. For example, some technology, while effective in reducing problem behavior under certain circumstances, may be difficult to implement within some community settings, thus limiting the generalizability of intervention effects. Long-term evaluation of the effectiveness of such technologies may bring to light supplemental intervention protocols that may be necessary to maintain success (e.g., teaching different communicative functions, fading or changing preferred items). Finally, social validity measures such as participant's preferences for assistive devices or other stakeholder evaluations (e.g., parents, teachers) of the practicality of the interventions may predict the success of such interventions.

References

Barlow, D. H., Nock, M. K., & Hersen, M. (2009). *Single case experimental designs: Strategies for studying behavior change* (3rd ed.). Boston: Allyn & Bacon.

Carr, E. G., & Smith, C. (1995). Biological setting events for self-injury. *Mental Retardation and Developmental Disabilities Research Reviews, 1*, 94–98.

Chadwick, O., Kusel, Y., & Cuddy, M. (2008). Factors associated with the risk of behavior problems in adolescents with severe intellectual disabilities. *Journal of Intellectual Disability Research, 52*, 864–876.

Cooper, S.-A., Smiley, E., Allan, L. M., Jackson, A., Finlayson, J., Mantry, D., & Morrison, J. (2009a). Adults with intellectual disabilities: Prevalence, incidence and remission of self-injurious behavior and related factors. *Journal of Intellectual Disability Research, 53*, 200–216.

Cooper, S.-A., Smiley, E., Jackson, A., Finlayson, J., Allan, L. M., Mantry, D., & Morrison, J. (2009b). Adults with intellectual disabilities: Prevalence, incidence and remission of aggressive behavior and related factors. *Journal of Intellectual Disability Research, 53*, 217–232.

Durand, V. M. (1993). Functional communication training using assistive devices: Effects on challenging behavior and affect. *Augmentative and Alternative Communication, 9*, 168–176.

Durand, V. M. (1999). Functional communication training using assistive devices: Recruiting natural communities of reinforcement. *Journal of Applied Behavior Analysis, 32*, 247–267.

Durand, V. M., & Crimmins, D. B. (1992). *The motivation assessment scale (MAS) administration guide*. Topeka: Monaco & Associates.

Emerson, E., & Einfeld, S. L. (2011). *Challenging behavior* (2nd ed.). New York: Cambridge University Press.

Emerson, E., Kiernan, C., Alborz, A., Reeves, D., Mason, H., Swarbrick, R., & Hatton, C. (2001). The prevalence of challenging behaviors: A total population study. *Research in Developmental Disabilities, 22*, 77–93.

Hanley, G. P., Iwata, B. A., & McCord, B. E. (2003). Functional analysis of problem behavior: A review. *Journal of Applied Behavior Analysis, 36*, 147–185.

Iwata, B. A., Dorsey, M. F., Slifer, K. J., Bauman, K. E., & Richlan, G. S. (1994). Toward a functional analysis of self-injury. *Journal of Applied Behavior Analysis, 27*, 197–209. (Reprinted from *Analysis and Intervention in Developmental Disabilities, 2*, 3–20, 1982).

Kahng, S., Iwata, B. A., & Lewin, A. B. (2002). Behavioral treatment of self-injury, 1964 to 2000. *American Journal on Mental Retardation, 107*, 212–221.

Kennedy, C. H., & Souza, G. (1995). Functional analysis and treatment of eye poking. *Journal of Applied Behavior Analysis, 28*, 27–37.

Lancioni, G. E., O'Reilly, M. F., & Basili, G. (1999). Review of strategies for treating sleep problems in persons with severe and profound intellectual or multiple disabilities. *American Journal on Mental Retardation, 104*, 170–186.

Lancioni, G. E., O'Reilly, M. F., Singh, N. N., Oliva, D., Scalini, L., Vigo, C. M., & Groeneweg, J. (2005a). Further evaluation of microswitch clusters to enhance hand response and head control in persons with multiple disabilities. *Perceptual and Motor Skills, 100*, 689–694.

Lancioni, G. E., O'Reilly, M. F., Singh, N. N., Sigafoos, J., Didden, R., Oliva, D., & Francesca, C. (2010). Two children with multiple disabilities increase adaptive object manipulation and reduce inappropriate behavior via a technology assisted program. *Journal of Visual Impairment and Blindness, 104*, 714–719.

Lancioni, G. E., Singh, N. N., O'Reilly, M. F., Oliva, D., Scalini, L., Vigo, C. M., & Groeneweg, J. (2004). Microswitch clusters to support responding and appropriate posture of students with multiple disabilities: Three case evaluations. *Disability and Rehabilitation, 26*, 501–505.

Lancioni, G. E., Singh, N. N., O'Reilly, M. F., & Sigafoos, J. (2009). An overview of behavioral strategies for reducing hand-related stereotypies of persons with severe to profound intellectual and multiple disabilities: 1995–2007. *Research in Developmental Disabilities, 30*, 20–43.

Lancioni, G., Singh, N., O'Reilly, M., Sigafoos, J., & Didden, R. (2012). Function of challenging behaviors. In J. Matson (Ed.), Functional assessment for challenging behaviors (pp. 45–64). New York: Springer.

Lancioni, G. E., Singh, N. N., O'Reilly, M. F., Sigafoos, J., Oliva, D., Gatti, M., & Groeneweg, J. (2008). A microswitch-cluster program to foster adaptive responses and head control in students with multiple disabilities: Replication and validation assessment. *Research in Developmental Disabilities, 29*, 373–384.

Lancioni, G. E., Singh, N. N., O'Reilly, M. F., Sigafoos, J., Oliva, D., Pidala, S., & Bosco, A. (2007). Promoting adaptive foot movements and reducing hand mouthing and eye poking in a boy with multiple disabilities through microswitch technology. *Cognitive Behavior Therapy, 36*, 85–90.

Lancioni, G. E., Singh, N. N., O'Reilly, M. F., Sigafoos, J., Oliva, D., Smaldone, A., & Groeneweg, J. (2011). Promoting mouth-drying responses to reduce drooling effects by persons with intellectual and multiple disabilities: A study of two cases. *Research in Developmental Disabilities, 32*, 477–482.

Lancioni, G. E., Smaldone, A., O'Reilly, M. F., Singh, N. N., & Oliva, D. (2005b). Automatic prompting to reduce persistent tongue protrusion in a woman with severe to profound mental retardation. *Perceptual and Motor Skills, 101*, 515–518.

Matson, J. L., Bamburg, J. W., Cherry, K. E., & Paclawskyj, T. R. (1999). A validity study of the Questions About Behavior Function (QABF) scale: Predicting treatment success for self-injury, aggression, and stereotypies. *Research in Developmental Disabilities, 20*, 163–175.

Matson, J. L., & Wilkins, J. (2009). Factors associated with the questions about behavior function for functional assessment of low and high rate challenging behaviors in adults with intellectual disability. *Behavior Modification, 33*, 207–219.

Murphy, G. H., Beadle-Brown, J., Wing, L., Gould, J., Shah, A., & Holmes, N. (2005). Chronicity of challenging behaviors in people with severe intellectual disabilities and/or autism: A total population sample. *Journal of Autism and Developmental Disorders, 35*, 405–418.

Oliver, C., Murphy, G. H., & Corbett, J. A. (1987). Self-injurious behavior in people with mental handicap: A total population study. *Journal of Mental Deficiency Research, 31*, 147–162.

Paclawskyj, T. R., Matson, J. L., Rush, K. S., Smalls, Y., & Vollmer, T. R. (2000). Questions About Behavioral Functions (QABF): A behavioral checklist for functional assessment of aberrant behavior. *Research in Developmental Disabilities, 21*, 223–229.

Poppes, P., van der Putten, A. J. J., & Vlaskamp, C. (2010). Frequency and severity of challenging behavior in people with profound intellectual and multiple disabilities. *Research in Developmental Disabilities, 31*, 1269–1275.

Qureshi, H., & Alborz, A. (1992). Epidemiology of challenging behavior. *Mental Handicap Research, 5*, 130–145.

Rojahn, J., Matson, J. L., Lott, D., Esbensen, A. J., & Smalls, Y. (2001). The Behavior Problems Inventory: An instrument for the assessment of self-injury, stereotyped behavior, and aggression/destruction in individuals with developmental disabilities. *Journal of Autism and Developmental Disorders, 31*, 577–588.

Saloviita, T. (2000). The structure and correlates of self-injurious behavior in an institutional setting. *Research in Developmental Disabilities, 21*, 501–511.

Sigafoos, J., Arthur, M., & O'Reilly, M. F. (2003). *Challenging behavior and developmental disability*. Baltimore: Paul H. Brookes Publishing Company.

Sigafoos, J., Elkins, J., Kerr, M., & Attwood, T. (1994). A survey of aggressive behavior among a population with intellectual disability in Queensland. *Journal of Intellectual Disability Research, 38*, 369–381.

Singh, A. N., Matson, J. L., Mouttapa, M., Pella, R. D., Hill, B. D., & Thorson, R. (2009). A critical item analysis of the QABF: Development of a short form assessment instrument. *Research in Developmental Disabilities, 30*, 782–792.

Steege, M. W., Wacker, D. P., Cigrand, K. C., Berg, W. K., Novak, C. G., Reimers, T. M., & DeRaad, A. (1990). Use of negative reinforcement in the treatment of self-injurious behavior. *Journal of Applied Behavior Analysis, 23*, 459–467.

Assistive Technology

Academic achievement
Ambulation
ASD
Assistive technology
Autism
Behavior management
Computer-based instruction
Daily living skills
Developmental disabilities
Education
Employment
Instructional technology
Learning
Leisure skills
Microswitches
Mobility
Multiple disabilities
Object-means
Occupational development
Occupational therapy
Orientation
Play
Recreation
Rehabilitation
Self-management
Social-emotional behavior
Speech-generating devices
Video modeling
Video prompting
Virtual reality
VOCAs
Voice-outcome communication aids

G.E. Lancioni et al., *Assistive Technology: Interventions for Individuals with Severe/Profound and Multiple Disabilities*, Autism and Child Psychopathology Series,
DOI 10.1007/978-1-4614-4229-5,

Index

G.E. Lancioni et al., *Assistive Technology: Interventions for Individuals with Severe/Profound and Multiple Disabilities*, Autism and Child Psychopathology Series, DOI 10.1007/978-1-4614-4229-5,

Printed by Printforce, the Netherlands